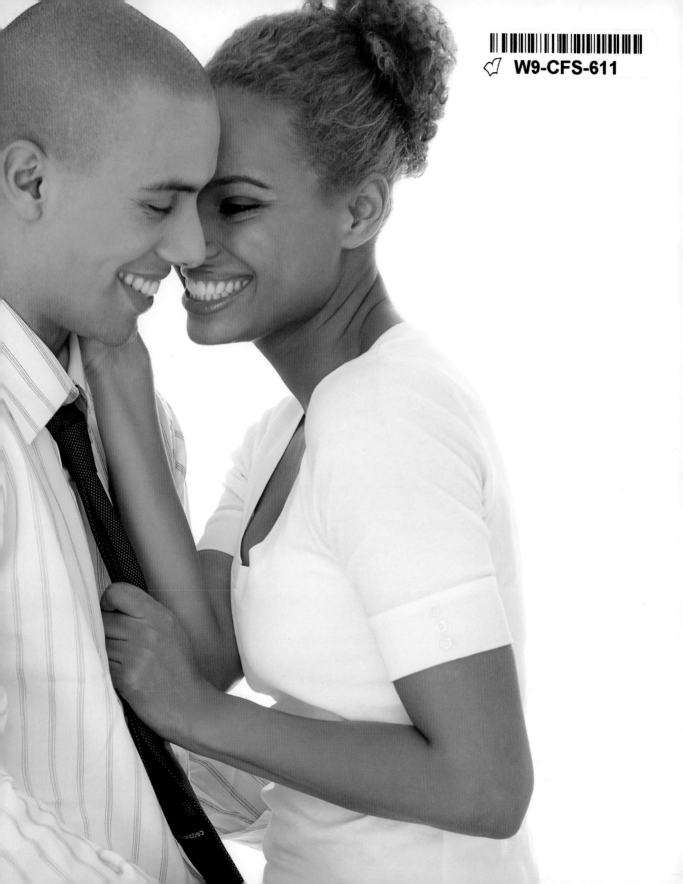

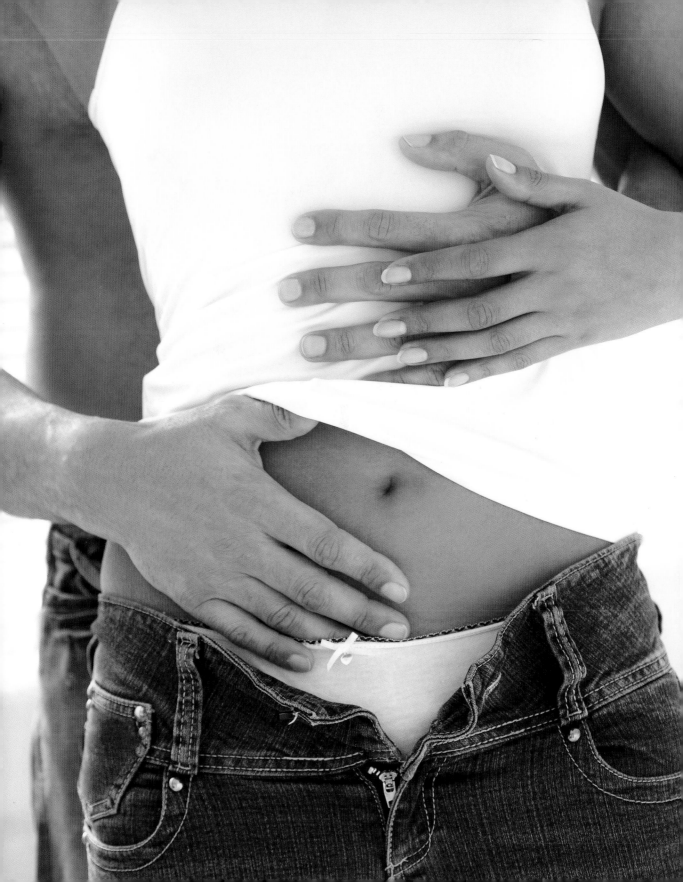

real sex
for real
women

intimacy, pleasure
& sexual well-being

Laura Berman PhD

Contents

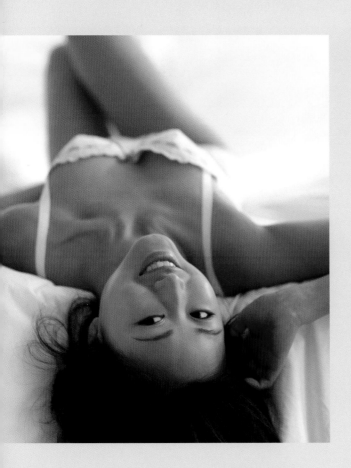

The quest for great sex

Sex is what separates lovers and friends. It is what makes a marriage more than just a partnership and parenthood. Sex fulfills our deep and natural need for intimacy and it bonds us with our partners in ways that are almost indefinable. Sex is something that we want, something that we need, and something that has the power to take us from stage one in a relationship to happily ever after.

In general, many of us feel that sex is a lot like pizza. No matter how bad it may be, it is still pretty good. However, those of us who have encountered a lackluster sex life know that lack of passion can kill a relationship. Even when everything else is on track—your careers are going smoothly, you and your partner are getting along swimmingly, the kids are happy—poor sexual pleasure can throw a wrench in your relationship dynamic.

That being said, great sex doesn't happen overnight, and if we were honest, most of us would have to admit that life is not always perfect between the sheets. Whether you aren't getting enough foreplay or you feel your partner isn't adventurous enough, there is probably something about your sex life that you would like to improve. How can a real woman—with real curves, a real career, and maybe even real parenting responsibilities— find practical advice for creating a youthful, joyful sexual relationship with her partner?

As a sex therapist and relationship counselor, I have spent two decades helping people with similar issues navigate the difficult world of sex and relationships. From young mothers to harried career women, my clients have run the gamut when it comes to age, family background, relationship status, profession, and individual needs. I have helped clients who were the victims of sexual abuse, clients who were in the middle of an affair, clients who didn't know the first thing about their own genital anatomy, and clients who were trying to figure out their own sexual orientation and sexual needs.

These experiences have taught me one important thing: we all need love and acceptance. We want our partners to cherish our bodies, crave our touch, and be fulfilled by our intimacy. We want to have passionate, no-holds-barred sex with our partner that leaves us feeling satiated, complete, and understood.

These are all emotional and physical needs which can and should be met in a happy, healthy relationship. All it takes is a little bit of knowledge and the willingness to stay committed to each other's needs and the improvement of the relationship as a whole. This book will guide you through that process, from helping you understand the brain chemicals that make men and women inherently different, to giving you tips and tricks for turning humdrum sex into orgasmic, fulfilling sex every time. From new positions to breathing techniques to a little bit of role-playing advice, this book is geared toward women who want to increase pleasure and confidence in every aspect of their lives.

I know that you're unbelievably busy. I know that some days you barely have time to eat a decent meal, let alone don complicated lingerie and cook a candlelit dinner for your partner. This book isn't going to ask you to do any of those things, unless you so desire. Instead, I'm going to help you figure out your own sexual needs and become acquainted with your own sexual potential. This book will help you finally create the sex life you've always wanted. Along the way, you might have to confront some of your fears and face down some of your insecurities, but the stories and advice in this book are from women just like you and will help you realize that you are not alone.

You can even use this book as a conversation starter with your partner. When you find something that piques your interest, whether it is a daring new position or an interesting bit of research, turn down the corner to show to your partner later. Let him be part of your journey to better sex—chances are, you won't have to ask him twice.

Now, let us begin our quest for great sex.

Laura Berman

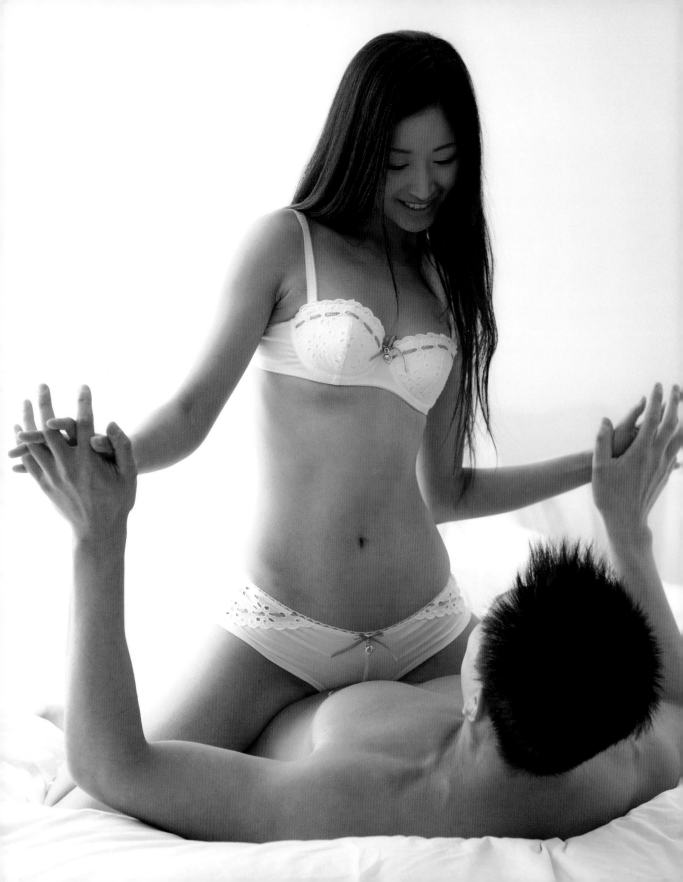

sex for life

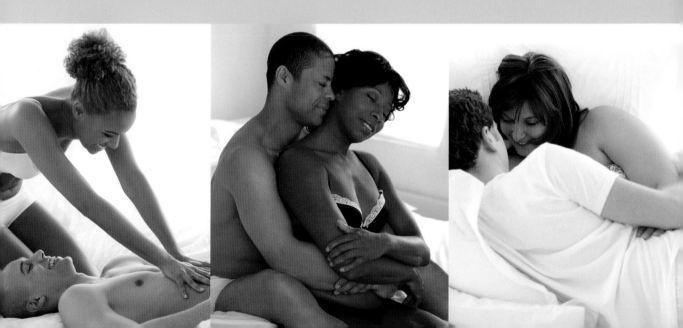

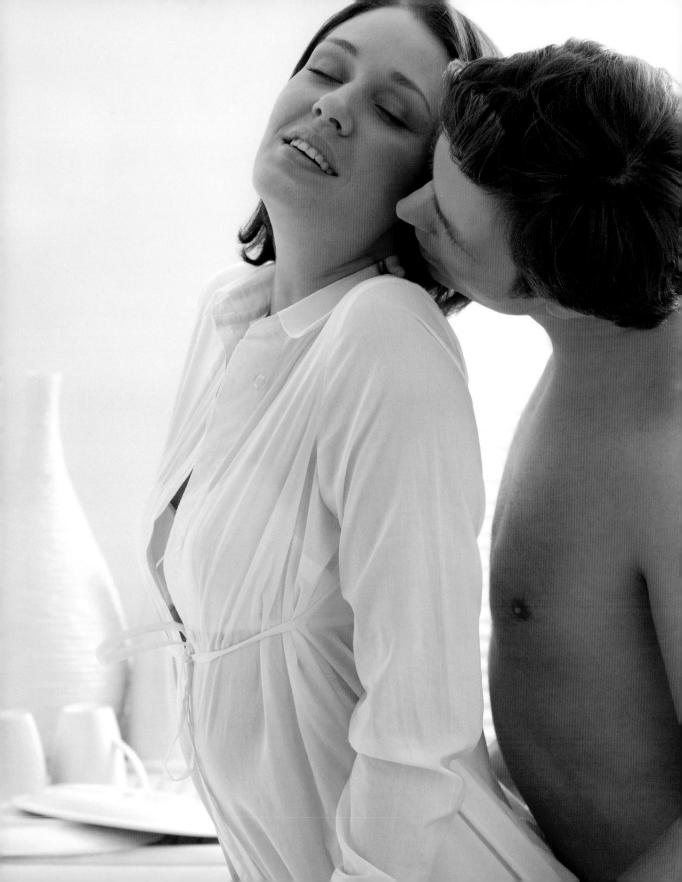

Sex matters

Sex is a fundamental part of humanity, and your sexuality is an essential part of your womanhood. Throughout life, sex is the driving force that creates energy, life, and attraction all around us. Learn how to harness your sexual energy and use it to become a creative and happy person. To deny our ties to sexuality and our need for sexual fulfilment is to deny our existence—sex is how we were created, and how we create. Understanding and accepting your sexuality will lead you to pleasure, confidence, and a fulfilling, intimate relationship with your lover. Celebrate sex, and you celebrate life.

Understanding sexuality

Whoever you are, whatever your circumstances or age, sex is vital to your emotional well-being, self-esteem, health, and relationships. Accepting your sexuality, and your partner's, puts you in charge of a very important part of your happiness—your physical satisfaction. Sexuality is rarely understood for what it truly is—an innate and healthy part of being alive and being human. It is actually our life force. Being comfortable with your sexuality is the first step on the road to a great sex—and love—life.

Human sexuality

Sexuality occurs long before adolescence. We are born sexual creatures—ultrasound scans have shown that male babies have erections as young as 16 weeks of age, and babies and children are inherently interested in their own bodies. Of course, we are not ready to be sexual at this young age. It is merely proof that sexuality is embedded in our genes; it is part of our being.

Your sexuality

If you understand your sexuality, you accept your sexual feelings, are able to express your desires to your lover, and find that sex adds intimacy to your relationship. Most importantly, you feel good about yourself. If you don't get enough sex you will feel its effects throughout your life in your health and emotions.

Even though sex is used to sell everything from chocolate and ice cream to cars and aftershave, we are less likely than the previous generation to be adventurous or sexually self-accepting. The problem is twofold: fear and media stereotypes. We fear the effects of too many sexual partners on our health, and are inhibited because we think that sex should look good rather than feel good.

Reviewing your sexual needs

Throughout your lifetime, and your relationship, your sexual needs evolve, often in response to your relationship status. A new baby, a new job, or a new partner can change your sexual desires considerably. It is important to take your life stage into account, and evaluate your needs.

What is certain is that you can't have a fulfilling sex life if you don't understand and accept each other's sexuality. Whatever your circumstances, staying in touch with each other by talking, touching, and kissing is vital, as is being able to talk openly and honestly about your sexual needs or desires. Take time to talk with your lover in bed, to play with different ideas and adventures, and enjoy being physically close.

Be brave

Don't let fear of change or the unknown hold you back. Tuning into your sexuality and having a healthy sex life is vital to your womanhood. Sex is as natural as breathing. Challenge any view that confines your sexuality and begin to fully understand your sexual desires and needs. Our sexuality is as fluid and diverse as the cultures on the Earth—an ever-evolving "sexual continuum."

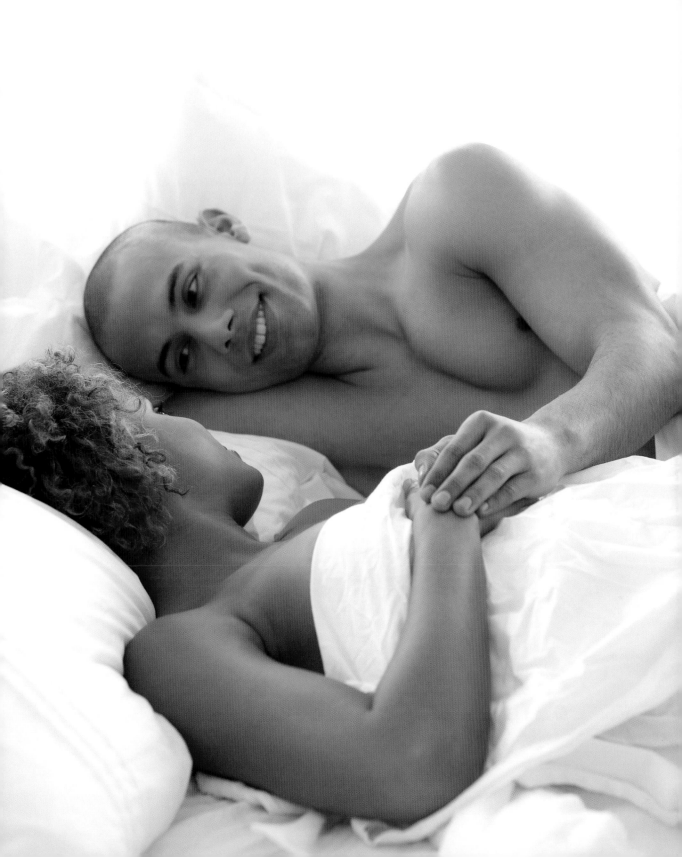

Female sexuality

Our sexuality is defined by who we are, and in turn, we are defined by our sexuality. A woman in touch with her sexuality feels confident, attractive, strong, and self-sufficient. Sex affects all areas of your relationship, not just in the bedroom. We were designed to be sexual creatures—divine divas who adore sexual pleasure, question sexual discontent, and strive for balance, harmony, and enjoyment. Your sexuality impacts the quality of your life, and developing a healthy sex life brings you happiness.

Sex and confidence

A fulfilling sex life enhances your self-esteem, relationships, and health, and also largely determines your happiness. Women who are confident and content with their sex life feel their confidence and contentment extend beyond the bedroom. The true "afterglow" of sex might be that you feel more beautiful and loved after a great session with your lover, and those positive feelings spur you on to greater achievements in your career and personal endeavors.

Your sexual needs

The problem is that some women don't put a high value on their sexuality. Male pleasure often takes precedence in the bedroom, and even the bravest of women may fear asking for something different or new from their partner. Women worry their partner might be offended or think they are being bossy and domineering; worse, they think their sexual demands suggest the exent of their experience in the bedroom. Consequently, some women never find out what arouses them. If you want to be sexually empowered focus on your own pleasure, too. A healthy sex life is one where both partners feel sexually satisfied.

Sexuality in the media

In your quest for your sexuality, look to yourself, your partner, and other inspirational females for the path. Women's magazines are often geared toward male pleasure and do little to empower women to seek their own orgasmic bliss. Scantily clad supermodels coupled with articles telling you how to please your partner only undermine your sexuality. After reading these articles, many

Women who are confident and content with their sex life feel their confidence and contentment extend beyond the bedroom.

women actually experience a decline in self-esteem. And nothing creates a roadblock to connecting with your sexual enjoyment like low self-esteem or having a poor body image.

Time to rediscover your sexuality

How can you get in touch with your sexuality? Break free from the media's erroneous definitions of sexuality. Don't worry that you are not the airbrushed sex goddess featured in lingerie commercials or movies—these images are designed to sell products, while your sexuality is boundless and unique. It doesn't matter that you don't have time to shave your legs every morning or energy to starve and sweat your way into a miniature-sized thong. The important thing, whoever you are, is to realize that you deserve a rewarding sex life—and that you can attain it.

Steps to a healthy sex life

If you want to reclaim your sexuality and enjoy a healthy sex life, you will need a few tools. Confidence in yourself is mandatory, so spend time caring for your body and finding out how it works. Get in touch with your sexual fantasies, then tell your partner—or even better, show him—what turns you on. A few new techniques will help you and your partner achieve heightened orgasms and intimacy. Embrace foreplay, oral sex, and fantasy play to enhance excitement in your sex life. All of this is covered in the chapters ahead, so read on to learn how to add these tricks to your sexual repertoire.

Your sexual needs evolve depending on your circumstances, and should be kept under review. In other words, if you and your partner are still making the same moves in your fifties that worked in your twenties, don't be surprised if your sex life is not as satisfying as it could be. Believe that your sexuality matters, devote time to making it as fulfilling as possible, and allow it to empower all of your life.

The benefits of sex

Regular sex is known to have six amazing health benefits: it increases youthful appearance, promotes the body's production of germ-fighting antibodies, strengthens the pelvic floor, burns calories, stabilizes the menstrual cycle, and gives natural pain relief through orgasms. Turns out great sex not only feels good, it keeps your relationship and personal life on track, and your body in tip-top shape. So go get some!

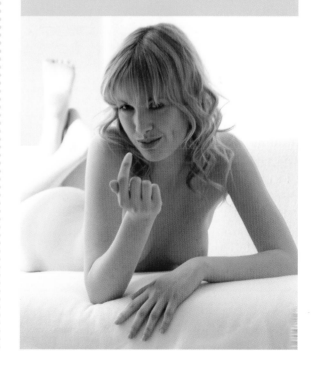

Male sexuality

Male sexuality is a bit of a mystery to women. According to the media, most men don't care who they have sex with, just as long as it feels good, and their lust is satisfied. The truth is quite different. Men have fewer sexual inhibitions and are less concerned about society's expectations of sex, but they have a very emotional connection to their sexuality. They are just as emotionally present and vulnerable during lovemaking as women. Women can learn from their positive attitude toward their sexuality.

Changing times

As women become more vocal about their sexual needs, men become more vocal about their emotional needs. This is good news for both men and women—by breaking out of their sexual stereotypes and embracing sexuality, couples feel free to express their desires to each other and create a more fulfilling and intimate sex life.

His emotional connection

So what contributes to a man's emotional connection during sex? The same things that you look for. A man needs to know that he is held in high esteem by his partner, that he is loved and needed. Arguments, lack of intimacy, and miscommunication all affect his sexuality. Keeping high levels of intimacy, talking to your man about his feelings, and making him feel good about himself will enhance your emotional and, consequently, sexual connection. So you both need to express your sexual desires.

This is important, because most men also need to know they are satisfying their partner. Sexual performance is a vital part of a man's self-esteem, and sexual longevity and prowess are key issues for most men. However, a man's need to satisfy his partner can sometimes create anxiety and tension in the bedroom—while he feels under pressure to be a great lover, his partner worries that she must have an orgasm to avoid hurting his feelings. Meanwhile, pressure to have an orgasm makes having one virtually impossible.

This type of tension in the bedroom is negative and stressful. Resolve this situation by letting your partner know that orgasm is not the be-all and end-all of your sexual experience. Tell him you

Men love sex. All of it—silk stockings and garters, red lipstick, uninhibited sounds and sights, its smell, and even the wet patch.

want to relax and enjoy the sensations. Let him know that it is not the orgasm but the intimacy and connection to the person she is having sex with that determines a woman's sexual satisfaction. Orgasm or not, reassure him that the experience will be pleasurable for you. Hopefully that will relieve him of his anxiety to satisfy you.

Media messages

Another little-known fact about male sexuality is that men struggle with body image issues, too. Women think they own the market when it comes to dieting woes and cellulite crises, but men are also likely to suffer from low self-esteem regarding their appearance. Surrounded by images of superheroes, muscle-bound billboard models, and the latest celebrity "It" guys, men are capable of self-doubt when they look down at their own not-so-rock-hard abs. As for below-the-belt body image: well, we know that size does matter—to men at least.

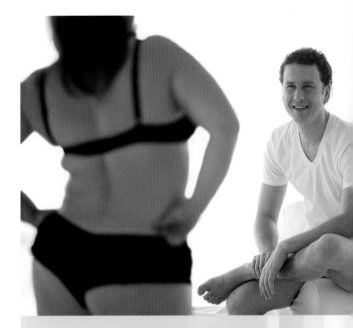

If your partner is feeling low about recent weight gain or suffering from locker-room envy over his anatomy, don't be surprised if his poor self-esteem spills over into the bedroom. Men need to hear that they are sexually attractive to their lover. The next time you wonder why your partner hasn't been as amorous lately, remind yourself to send a few compliments his way.

Learn from his type of sexuality

Men love sex. In all its gore and its glory—silk stockings, red lipstick, uninhibited sounds and sights, its musky smell, and even sleeping in the wet patch. Your man's ability to experience sex with uninhibited enjoyment is a valuable lesson to take from his unique sexuality. But role-play, new positions, and learning new ways to pleasure each other can be a freeing experience for both of you. Understanding each other's sexuality will bring renewed intimacy and passion to your emotional and physical lives.

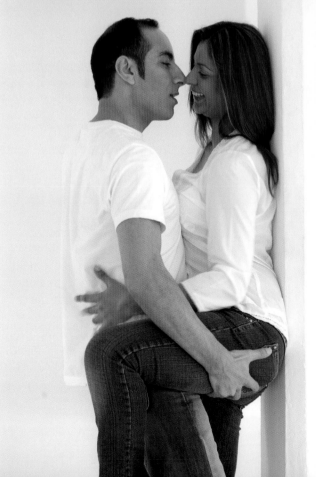

Male and female sexual differences

When it comes to sex, men and women often have very different opinions about what goes on in the bedroom—from how often is enough, to which position is best, to favorite time of day or night to make love. Luckily, we agree on one thing—sex feels great. Sexuality is unique to each individual and there are many contributing factors that affect how and when we want sex. These include lifestyle factors, arousal needs, gender differences, and even our evolutionary ties to sex and relationships.

Sexual roles and monogamy

Since the earliest Homo sapiens, the success of the human race has depended on the ability of men to spread their genes as far as possible. The more sexual partners they had, the more likely it was that their genes would pass on to the next generation. It did not benefit women to have sex with the whole tribe, however—they only needed to have sex with the man who could help them survive pregnancy and beyond. Women were driven to mate with the most powerful male in the group, since he offered the greatest protection.

These sexual differences between men and women still hold true today. Men tend to boast about their number of sexual partners, whereas women are more reluctant to disclose theirs. In addition, it is female sex drive that possibly created the beginnings of monogamy. The woman would pledge fidelity to the male so that he could be assured that the baby she had would be his. He would then commit to stay with her and provide for her during pregnancy and childhood. These monogamy "contracts" are thought to have been temporary, as in serial monogamy, in which a person has many monogamous relationships throughout their lifetime.

Arousal factors

Women have strong physical ties to sexuality, but we don't have sex like men. When a man sees a sexy image—such as their partner bending over to clean the bath or a glimpse of her naked flesh—he is aroused and may respond by pressing himself against her and wanting sex urgently. Women can also be aroused by visual stimuli, but tend to need more kinesthetic ones—such as stroking, kissing, and cuddling—to reach a point of wanting to have sex.

Men love the immediacy of arousal and the seduction of their woman into the bedroom. Women, on the other hand, tend to enjoy the prolonged intimacy of cuddling, stroking, and kissing. Men tend to wake up with an erection, whereas women tend to prefer nighttime sex after they have relaxed, or had a bath.

Multi-tasking and sex

Women take longer to become aroused and achieve orgasm because we are not as goal-oriented as men. Women's brains have evolved to be more adapted to multitasking, and this means we cannot zoom from zero to 50 in under five minutes. While our multitasking skills allow us to be superwomen for our families, it also means that enjoying sex can be a bit of a struggle for us. It is harder for us to detach from our worries and simply enjoy sex. More often than not, we are thinking about the kids' homework, the laundry, the dishes, or the big meeting at work the next day. Men find it easier to disengage from their worries and revel in the pleasures of sex, which is why it is important for our partners to understand that we need foreplay and extra time to enjoy sex.

These different sexual needs can sometimes lead to relationship problems, primarily because neither partner understands the other's needs. It helps to be honest about your differences. Be straightforward and tell your lover you crave more foreplay, a new position, or more sex—and then ask him what he craves. He probably has a few needs of his own that aren't being met.

The gender-switch generation
Changing gender roles challenges many couples to rethink their place in the relationship. For instance, men who earn less than their partner, or men who work as the homemaker, can have a hard time finding their footing in the bedroom.

In addition, one of the most significant trends is gender confusion among women. In today's corporate world the last thing women want to show is any type of weakness or emotion. This attitude can carry over into her personal relationships. But too much control in the bedroom is not a good thing for your sex life. Men need to feel sexually in charge some of the time, just as you do.

An empowered woman is confident enough in her own mind to allow her man to make some of the decisions and share in the control.

As gender roles in our society shift and evolve, couples should be prepared for a little backlash in the bedroom—but with compromise and equality on both sides of the relationship, sex can actually improve in these empowered waters.

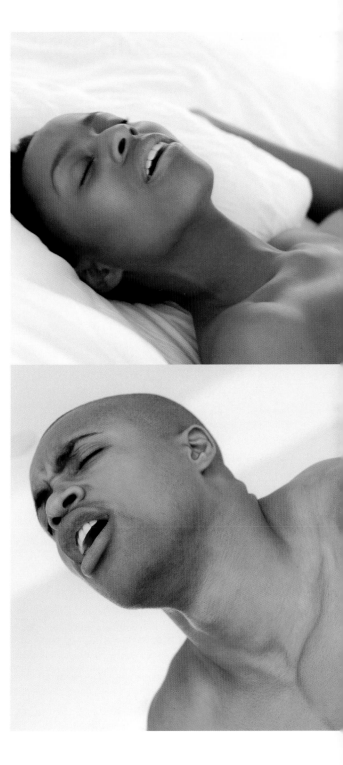

Sex and intimacy

Intimacy is the fiber that binds us to the people we love, and is built on time, investment, and honest communication. In a healthy long-term relationship, intimacy increases with time and many men and women are fortunate to have a lover who is also their best friend. Sex and romance are crucial for long-term intimacy. The stronger the sexual connection, the stronger the emotional intimacy will be. It is important to nurture and feed your relationship both emotionally and sexually.

The sex and intimacy cycle

Sex and intimacy are closely linked in our brains, but men and women respond differently to intimacy. Many men can't feel intimate with their partner unless their sex life is satisfying, but many women can't enjoy sex without intimacy. For men, sex feeds intimacy, and for women, intimacy feeds sex. These sexual differences can be disruptive to your relationship so it is important to nourish your sex life with intimacy.

First love to familiarity

When you first met your lover, chances are you were overwhelmed with sensations of excitement, bliss, and smoldering desire. When you fall in love, your brain releases chemicals such as serotonin, adrenaline, and oxytocin. These chemicals create feelings of excitement and passion. As time goes by, and you become more comfortable together, your desire wanes and you stop having as much sex. This phase also tends to involve a loss of spark.

This happens because, over time, your brain becomes accustomed to these chemicals and requires more hormone to create the initial high. In other words, ongoing intense sexual excitement in a loving relationship goes against our biological instincts. This means you have to work at keeping the intimacy and attraction between you.

Obstacles to intimacy

When you or your partner are having a hard time—for example, at work—your poor mood will affect you both. Similarly, if your sex life is floundering, you will both feel the effects in all parts of your relationship. To keep intimacy in your relationship, you need to have a fulfilling sex life, and vice versa. Nourish your intimacy levels by making sure that you keep a physical connection alive—touching, kissing, and even talking will enhance your bond and intimacy.

The deepest and most fulfilling intimacy springs from the closeness of a long-term relationship and time spent keeping passion in your relationship. But if you have been with your partner for a long time, you may discover that you no longer have a high sex drive or get that little "zing" every time you kiss him or he touches you. There are many ways to reignite this spark and keep your sex life intimate and passionate. So get comfortable and keep reading.

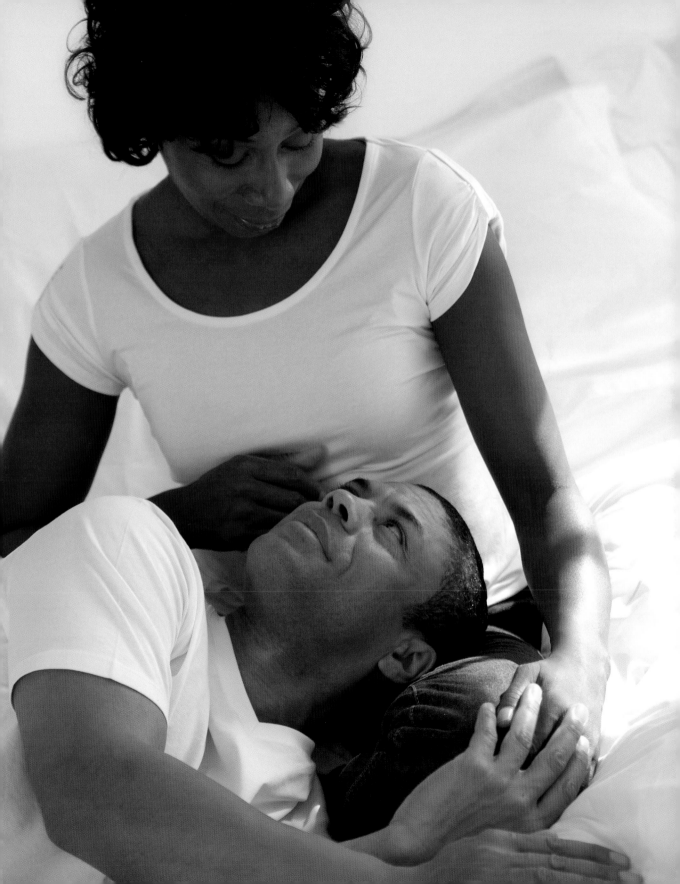

Making time for sex

How often have you collapsed into bed and fallen asleep exhausted not from a night of passion but from a too-full day of running around trying to take care of everything you need to do? For women especially, achieving a fulfilling sex life is about finding time: time to be intimate with your lover, time for yourself, and time to think about what you want from your sex life. To reinvigorate your relationship, try reassessing your priorities and making time to let sexiness flourish in your life.

Doing it all

The trouble with women is that we pride ourselves on doing it all. Even though we excel at working a double shift—holding down a full-time job then coming home to housework, cooking, and raising children—we find it hard to relax and enjoy life. To make matters worse, we often refuse help because we believe only we can do it right. Even when given the opportunity to relax, we often choose to spend the time packing lunches, answering emails, or writing a mental to-do list.

Life-enhancing time off

It might not be your partner or children that are stopping you from making time for sex—instead, it might be juggling commitments at work, at home, and with friends. Time for yourself will reward you with greater productivity and improve your relationships with colleagues and friends. Whatever its source, lack of sleep, stress, and a busy lifestyle cause many women to experience fatigue, weight gain, moodiness, and low sex drive. So the next time you're running ragged all day, don't be surprised if you head to bed feeling as sexy as a turnip.

You might not be sure where or how discovering your sexuality is supposed to fit into your busy life. But accept that you need time to rest and recuperate. If, like many women, you place sex at the bottom of your to-do list, it might be time to review your priorities and make time for sex. In order to have the best relationship and sex life possible, start by following the three Ds—delegate, decrease, and disengage—to overcome stress, and find time to enhance sex and intimacy with your partner.

If, like many women, you place sex at the bottom of your to-do list, it might be time to review your priorities to make time for sex in your life.

Delegate: extend your time

Mounting, nagging to-do lists drive us—and our partners—crazy, and we aren't doing anyone any favors by trying to do it all. Our bosses and co-workers are deprived of a calm colleague, our kids of a relaxed mother, our partners and our friends of spending quality time with us. We are deprived of energy, liveliness, and rest.

Prioritize your tasks. If you have a to-do list that includes more than five or six items, it is time to rethink. Put dates against tasks, and stars against anything you cannot delegate. Cross out nonessential tasks.

Your delegation operation might involve a monthly cleaning service. Housekeeping services are quite affordable, so let go of the reins and hand over the mop. Meanwhile, you will have gained an hour of rest and recuperation, which will boost your mood and your libido.

Use technology to make your life easier. Order your groceries, birthday presents, and household items online. Save shopping trips for when you want to choose some sexy new underwear.

Decrease: simplify

How do you decrease? Take a deep breath and let go of perfection. Okay, so there are crumbs on the kitchen table—the world is not going to end. Barring a major bug problem, it should be safe for you to go to sleep at night without sweeping up every crumb in the house.

Make your life easier wherever and whenever possible. From dishwashers to prepackaged meals to self-cleaning shower gadgets, there are a large number of products that will save you time and sweat. Some of them might be costly, but if they save you time in the end, they are worth it.

You will also have to learn to say "no" more often. Set up boundaries to protect your emotional and physical well-being. Cut back on the number of committees you join, and don't agree to host every family function or holiday party at your

Share the load

Talk to your partner about sharing a few of the household chores—maybe he won't do them as you would, but the laundry gets done and the beds made. Delegate a few home responsibilities to your kids, if you have them. Most children like being given responsibility. Simple chores like setting the table, dusting, and pairing socks, are easy ways to get the whole family involved in the business of running the house.

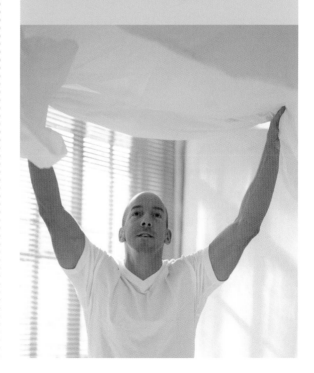

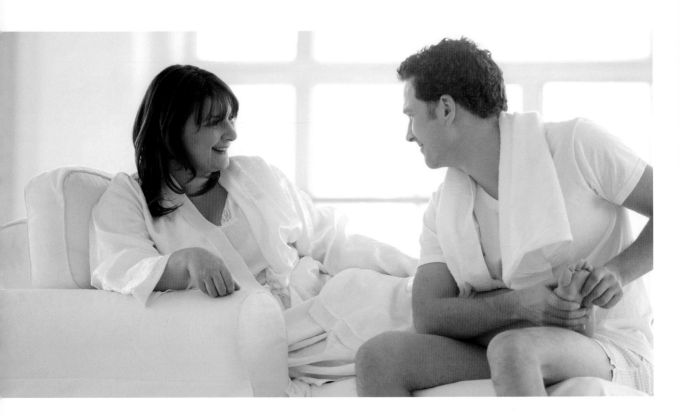

house. Most people will respect your decision. It is nice to feel needed, but resolve to trim down your social obligations, and save yourself for only those that you truly enjoy. The same goes for your kids' activities. Save your, and their, energy for the ones they can't live without or give up. Use the time to relax with your feet up. To reclaim your sex life back you need "your" time back.

Disengage: reconnect with you

Have you ever booked a massage then spent the time worrying about the weird noise your car is making? Or desperately wanted to go to sleep only to find your mind racing because you aren't able to turn off the adrenaline rushing through your body? For many women, a lack of time isn't the only problem—we find it hard to relax, too, even when we do have a few moments to ourselves.

This is where exercise is helpful. A brisk walk, a session in the gym, a swim, even digging in the garden will get your heart pumping and your hormones flowing. The result is that you'll feel energized and relaxed. If that sounds like too much activity, yoga is a less energetic relaxation tool. While doing the exercises, you are only able to think of the poses at hand—and not the million things left on your to-do list. Any type of exercise that encourages you to slow down and focus on your breathing will help you relax. When you focus on controlling your breath, you are too preoccupied to focus on mundane worries.

Take five minutes every day to sit calmly, breathe deeply and calm your mind. Breathe in through your mouth and out through your nose. Use this deep-breathing technique to relax your body and mind whenever you feel stressed.

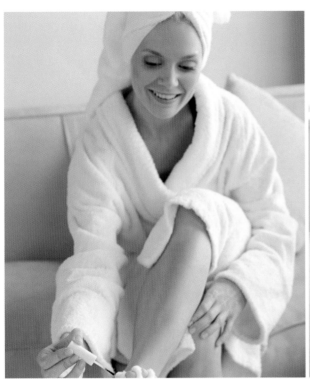
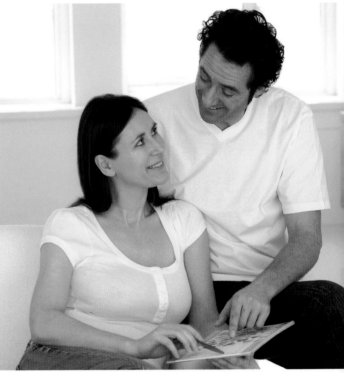

Quit waiting for the perfect life

We are always seeking perfection, whether it is in our looks, our careers, or our families. We want to rest and relax—but only after everything else in our lives is perfect. Have you ever thought to yourself: I will spend more time on my marriage when the kids are in college. I will devote myself to my own needs once my finances are more settled. I will get into shape when the children go to school—the list is endless. What are you waiting for? What personal happiness or fulfilment are you delaying for perfection? Now is the absolute best time to seek your own happiness.

What does this mean? It means stop living for the future and live for today. It means you don't need to be thinner and more toned to have a fantastic sex life with your partner. And don't delay your happiness until some non-existent utopia finds you. Focus on the present, and enhance your time and life now rather than always working toward tomorrow.

Rediscover your single self

This doesn't mean you should leave your partner. It means finding time to reconnect with the woman you used to be—the one your partner fell in love with. Make time for old interests, forgotten girlfriends, and grooming rituals. Take long walks through the woods or along the shore. Have a spa or beauty treatment. Look at photographs of yourself and your partner and reminisce about when you first met. Lie down and daydream about having sex just the way you want it. Activities such as these recharge your independence and reconnect you to your femininity—things we often lose track of in the stress of day-to-day life.

Sex files: Making time for sex

Between working hard, raising children, and all your other commitments it can seem impossible to find time for your relationship. But your love life is a living organic thing that needs emotional and sexual intimacy to flourish. Here's how one couple changed their priorities to find time for sex.

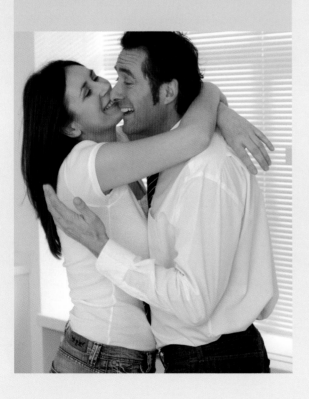

Background

Danielle, 35 years old, is an insurance agent for a large company, and her husband Frank, 37, runs a computer business. Danielle works up to 60 hours a week and, apart from the time she took to have children, she's never had an extended break from work. She also works hard at being a mom. Before having children, Danielle and Frank had sex four or five times a week.

The problem

Danielle and Frank were locked into arguments, usually about money and time constraints. Frank wanted Danielle to cut back on her hours at work, but Danielle felt they wouldn't be able to manage on less money. Danielle had lost all interest in sex. "After I gave birth to Jessie and then Mark, my interest in sex plummeted. Between a full-time career and caring for the kids, the last thing on my mind was sex."

Frank felt he was getting more and more detached from Danielle because she never had any time for him. He told me: "I miss Danny and I miss sex. Danny thinks she has to do everything—work, kids, housework—I wish she'd let go a bit."

Finding solutions

I talked at length to Danielle about her priorities in life. We discussed her attitudes to work, her kids, and Frank. She began to realize that time spent at home with Frank and the children would be more valuable to her than money in the bank. As a first step to solving her relationship problems, Danielle decided to cut back on the number of hours she spent at work.

Next, I asked Danielle to make an inflexible, must-keep appointment in which she would spend five hours a week on "me" time. This could be having her nails done, watching television, going for a walk, reading a book, or taking a nap. I told Frank to hold her to this weekly appointment and to accept no excuses!

For their couples' assignment, I asked Danielle and Frank to plan a romantic getaway. Like so many parents, Danielle and Frank had not been on a kids-free vacation since Jessie and Mark were born. Although family trips build great memories, parents also need adult-only breaks in which they can get out of parenting mode and back into being partners and lovers. I hoped that Frank and Danielle would rediscover each other as individuals.

Last but not least, I asked Frank and Danielle to spend "alone" time together every day. This could simply be sharing a glass of wine or talking over a meal. I told them not to worry if sex didn't happen right away; my main aim was to get them sharing time and connecting emotionally again.

What happened?

Frank was delighted that Danielle reduced her working hours. They both made a commitment to take more care of their relationship and they strictly honored the "alone" time ritual. Danielle's desire to have sex developed slowly as her emotional bond with Frank grew. Having an adult-only break definitely helped their sexual reunion. They even made a pact to have sex once a week, whether it be a quickie in the morning before the kids got up, or a longer session on the weekend. And for the rest of the week they worked at creating a sexual spark. "Even a long goodbye kiss on the lips can make us feel special," said Danielle.

Dedicated "us" time

If you lead a hectic life, make the effort to spend a little time each day connecting with your partner. Even if you're not in the mood for sex, lie down and cuddle or have a light-hearted, teasing conversation. Don't fall into the trap of talking about work or domestic issues.

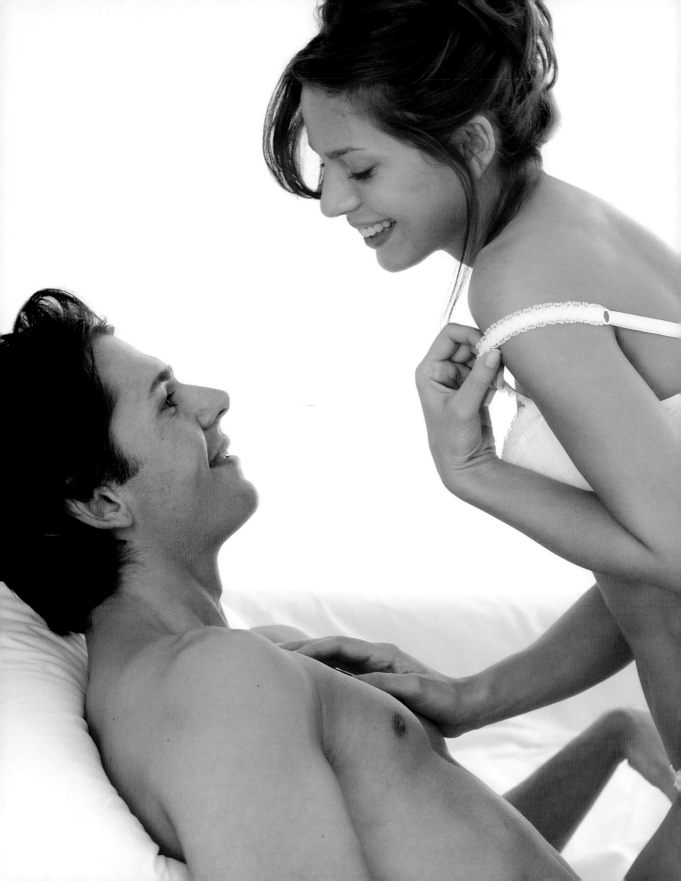

the sex
connection

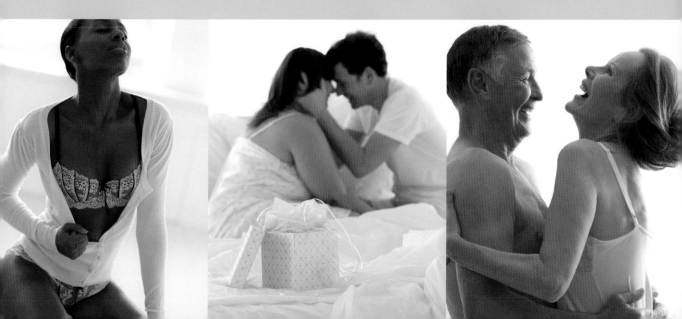

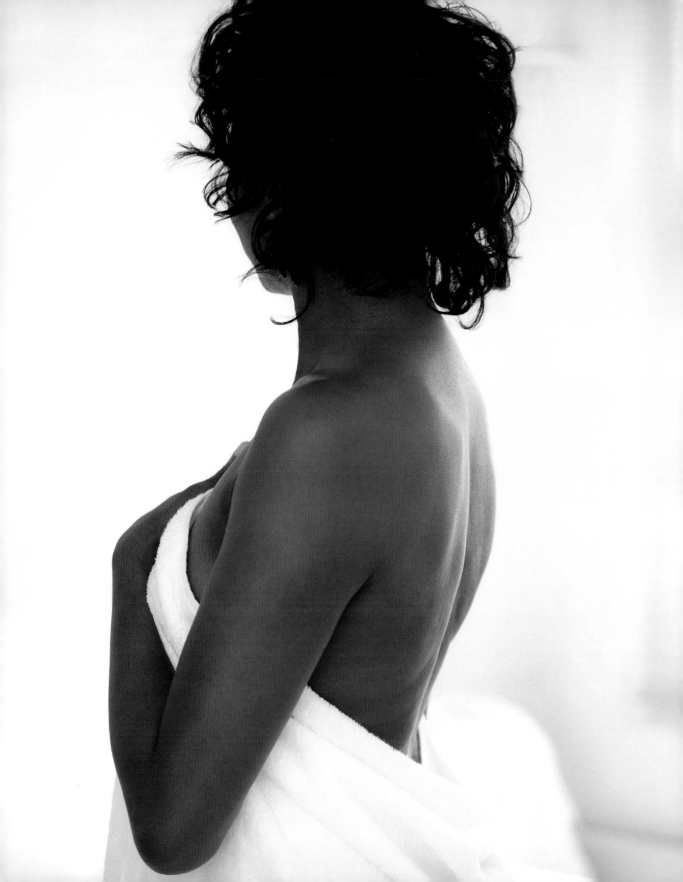

Know your body

To get in tune with your sexuality, you first need to connect with your body and appreciate the beauty of your womanhood, inside and out. Embracing your unique physical attributes, your shape and size, is vital for truly uninhibited and abandoned sex. Fears and anxieties about your body will only hold you back. A clear understanding of how your sexual responses work will help, and a positive genital self-image will enhance your love life. Self-knowledge and effective techniques for self-pleasure will also teach you what stimulation you need from your sex life, and how to get it.

Anatomy and sexual response

When tuning in to your sexuality, it is helpful to familiarize yourself with your genitals and their appearance. Begin by looking at them straight on. This might sound a bit intimidating, but is actually a very sexy thing to do—your genitals are a beautiful and natural part of your sexuality. The first step to a healthy sex life is a good anatomy lesson: get to know the dimensions of your genitals, and explore how different areas respond to stimulation. Knowledge is power, so let us apply that power to sex.

Feel good about yourself

The idea of loving your genitals might sound silly, but if you are insecure about them, you will have a hard time embracing your sexuality and being uninhibited in the bedroom. Men and women alike may suffer from genital self-esteem issues, but the good news is that dealing with these issues will vastly improve your sex life.

A woman who feels good about her genitals is six times more likely to be sexually satisfied than a woman who does not—if you don't like your own genitals, chances are you won't be able to let go and enjoy yourself when your partner is up close and personal with them.

Men also experience anxieties about their penises, worrying that they might be too small, too big, or too curved. A man has a strong emotional connection to his penis, so when he is comfortable with the way it looks and feels, he is more likely to be relaxed during sex.

Rediscover your genitals

You may think you know all about your genitals, but it is important to reconnect with them at different stages of your adult life, as childbirth and advancing age can change the way you look and feel. Educating yourself will help you to overcome any fears you might have about touching yourself or being touched.

Looking at your genitals gives you the perfect opportunity to explore them. And as you get to know them, you will learn how they govern your sexual response. This doesn't just mean knowing where to find—and how to stimulate—your hot spots. It is about having a healthy emotional relationship with your genitals, and getting the most out of your sex life as a result.

Practice makes perfect

A healthy sexual response is also linked to having regular lovemaking sessions with your partner. The mantra "If you don't use it, you lose it" holds true for genital health. If you don't engage in regular sex or masturbation, your genital circulation suffers and your sexual response decreases. So the more you have sex, the more you should expect to enjoy it, since healthy circulation equals stronger, more intense orgasms.

Regular sessions in bed are good for your partner's sexual response as well—he will be able to last longer during lovemaking and benefit from more intense orgasms, too.

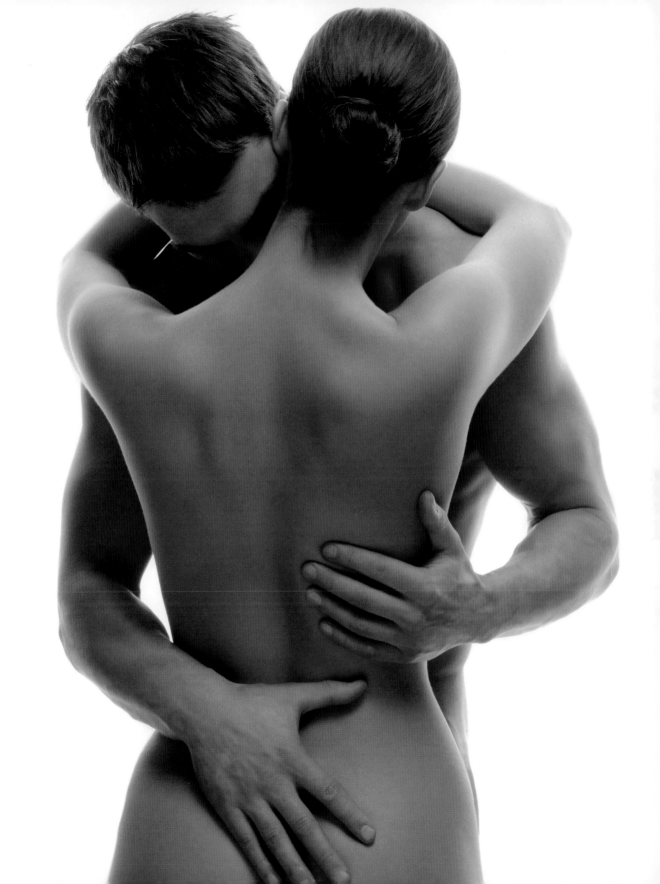

Female anatomy

The female anatomy is highly complex, deeply sensitive, and entirely beautiful. However, it is also subject to many common misconceptions. For instance, the vagina is just one part of a woman's sexual anatomy and most of the external anatomy is covered by the term "vulva." And what's all the fuss about the clitoris, anyway? There's no better way of clearing up any confusion than by taking a good look for yourself. So grab a hand-held mirror and spend some time identifying your many wonderful parts.

Mons pubis

The first thing you will see is the mons pubis, which is otherwise known as the mound of Venus. This is the small mass of flesh that sits above your genitals, on top of your pubic bone, and is usually covered with hair. Consisting of fatty tissue just beneath the skin, it helps protect the pubic bone.

Labia majora

These are the external female genitalia, also known as the outer labia or "lips." They are fleshy and rich in blood vessels and nerve endings. As with most women, your two labia majora will probably be of different sizes, like your breasts.

Many women enjoy having their labia rubbed, stroked, touched, and licked. When aroused, the labia fill with blood and become swollen, causing your genitals to tighten on your partner's penis.

Labia minora

The labia minora, or inner labia, are smaller folds of skin, which surround the vaginal opening and clitoris. They are very sensitive to touch and oral stimulation. When aroused, the labia minora secrete sebum, which lubricates the vagina.

The labia minora come in many different colors, sizes, and shapes, and this is completely natural, healthy, and even sexy.

Labiaplasty—a form of cosmetic surgery to trim and reshape a woman's labia majora and minora—is becoming increasingly popular, as some women fear that their labia are imperfect or deformed in some way. This surgery is not necessary or advisable, since it is possible that the labia's nerve endings may suffer damage during the procedure, which will have the effect of reducing your sexual response.

The Holy Grail of female sexual pleasure is the clitoris. It is filled with sensitive nerve endings, which feel wonderful when stimulated.

Clitoris

The Holy Grail of female sexual pleasure is the clitoris. Developed from the same tissue as the sensitive glans of the penis, the clitoris is located at the top of the vaginal entrance, inside the labia. It looks like a tiny pink nose. The clitoris is filled with sensitive nerve endings, which feel wonderful when stimulated.

The clitoris consists of three crucial parts. First are the clitoral crura, which are an internal portion of the clitoris. About 10 to 12 centimeters in length, the crura are like legs and reach back into the pelvis, almost to the pubic bone. They fill with blood when a woman becomes aroused. The clitoral head (otherwise known as the glans) is roughly the size and shape of a small pea, and is located near the very top of the labia. It is perhaps the most sensitive part of the clitoris, as it is filled with many rich nerve endings—more than any other part of the body, apart from the lips. The clitoral shaft is located down toward the vagina and then splits to each side into the crura. It is not visible to the naked eye since it is covered by a layer of skin and tissue.

Many women prefer their clitoris to be stimulated indirectly—through material or the labia—rather than via direct pressure, since it is often a super-sensitive part of their anatomy.

Urethra and periurethral sponge

This is the tube that stems from the bladder and releases your urine flow. If you have ever suffered from a urinary tract infection, you probably learned that the pain and burning is a result of bacteria getting into the urethra. The female urethra is shorter than the male urethra, which makes women more susceptible to these uncomfortable infections.

Surrounding the urethra is the periurethral sponge, which is also rich in nerve endings. Many women find it arousing to stimulate the area around the urethra.

Internal female anatomy

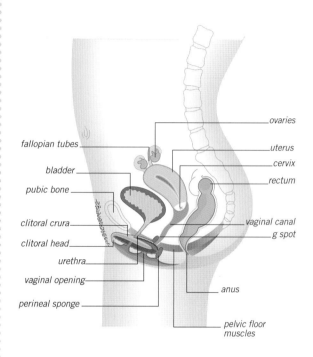

ovaries
fallopian tubes
bladder
pubic bone
clitoral crura
clitoral head
urethra
vaginal opening
perineal sponge
uterus
cervix
rectum
vaginal canal
g spot
anus
pelvic floor muscles

External female anatomy

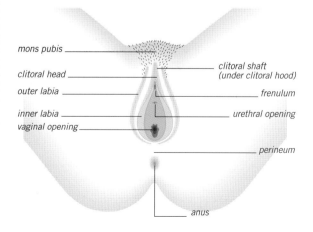

mons pubis
clitoral head
outer labia
inner labia
vaginal opening
clitoral shaft (under clitoral hood)
frenulum
urethral opening
perineum
anus

Vaginal opening

The entrance to the vagina—and its most visible part—the vaginal opening feels wonderful when gently rubbed. Around 30 percent of women are afflicted by vaginal or vulvar pain; those who suffer from the condition called vulvodyina experience a stinging, burning or itching sensation in this area, besides other external and internal discomfort and pain. The cause is uncertain, but could be related to allergies, diet, medication, or infections. If you suffer from any sort of pain in this area, seek medical advice.

Vagina

This is the canal that your partner's penis penetrates during sex, and through which a baby exits the uterus during childbirth. The vagina is a wonder of nature in that it can stretch to let a baby out, and yet is still small enough to tighten around a finger. Stronger vaginal muscles lead to better orgasms, but only the first third of the vagina is sensitive—good news for men who worry their penis is not large enough to please.

G-spot

Although some people debate its existence, the G-spot is real, and stimulating it can lead to heady sexual pleasure. It is located about two inches inside your vagina. To find it, insert a finger and hook it toward your belly button, as if gesturing for someone to come closer. You will find a spongy bump that some women compare to feeling the tip of their nose. When the G-spot is stimulated, you might feel an urge to urinate—one way of knowing you've found it. This feeling generally passes. The G-spot responds to a build-up of pressure from a finger, sex toy, or penis.

Cervix

Your cervix sits at the top of the vagina, or the bottom of the uterus. It has a tiny opening, which allows male sperm to pass in, and other fluids to pass out, such as blood during menstruation. During childbirth the diameter of the cervix expands to around four inches to allow the baby to descend into the vagina.

When a woman is aroused, her cervix lengthens and moves farther into the body to allow deeper penetration. Some women enjoy having their cervix stimulated by their partner's penis. You'll probably need to be fully aroused for this, but it can lead to a breathtaking orgasm.

Cervical health is vital to your well-being, and having regular cervical pap smears can protect your fertility, and save your life.

Perineum and perineal sponge

The perineum is located between the vaginal opening and the anus. It is filled with tiny nerve endings, which feel wonderful when pleasured. The perineal sponge, which is located underneath the perineum, is also filled with numerous nerve endings, and many women find it very arousing when pressure is applied to this area.

Fertility: uterus and internal organs

Your uterus (or womb) is a pear-shaped organ between your bladder and rectum. When you have an orgasm, the muscle lining of the uterus contracts, giving you a deep sensation of pleasure.

The inner layer of the uterus, known as the endometrial tissue, sheds every month after puberty (except during pregnancy and, usually, for some months after delivery for mothers who are breast-feeding.) This is what makes up the menstrual flow. Many women find regular orgasms can alleviate menstrual cramps, but do not delay in seeking medical advice if you have severe menstrual pain or abnormal periods.

Your ovaries are on either side of the uterus. These produce your primary female hormones, estrogen and progesterone. They also hold eggs, or ova. Each woman is born with about a million eggs, which are released regularly until menopause. An egg is moved from the ovary and along the fallopian tube by the fimbria—tiny hair-like structures with flared ends. If the egg is not fertilized, it disintegrates and passes out during menstruation. If it is fertilized, it attaches to the endometrial lining of the uterus and starts the amazing process of developing into an embryo.

Self care

Along with self-knowledge comes good self care. Some women go to lengths to clean their genitals, often at the risk of harm. The vagina has a delicate pH system, which is affected by douching, scented feminine wipes, and other perfumed products. Some cleaning products may cause infection. Even antibiotics can lead to vaginal yeast infections, such as thrush, since they kill the good bacteria that help the vagina stay healthy.

Your vagina is self-cleaning—it does not need any extra help to be deliciously fragrant and clean. A little warm water and mild soap on the external labia is all that is required. Vaginal odor is normal, and many men find it to be quite a turn-on. That said, if you notice a strange or new odor, or if the odour is so strong that you can smell it when naked, it could be a sign of an infection. In this case you should seek medical advice.

All women have different aesthetic preferences for their genital region—some prefer no pubic hair (known as a Brazilian), some prefer a small line left on the vulva, while others prefer a light trim to keep the hair manageable. Just make sure any products you use are hypo-allergenic. If you are having your hair removed at a salon, check that it is licensed for genital hair removal.

Kegel exercises will help maintain vaginal tone and function. Throughout the day, tense the muscles that lie in a figure-eight pattern around your vagina and anus—this will strengthen your pelvic floor and recreate tightness you may have lost due to childbirth, age, or other factors.

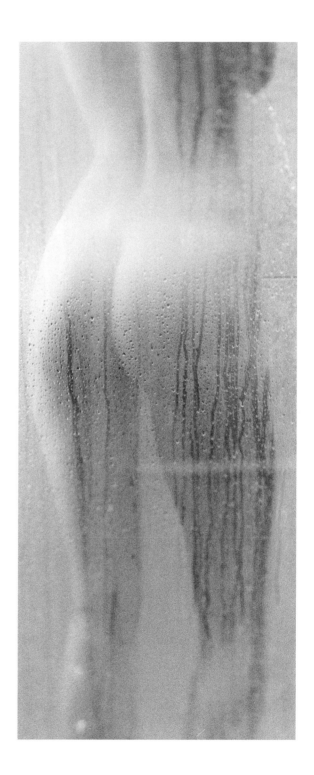

Male anatomy

The male anatomy might appear pretty straightforward, but even the most well-versed woman could use a refresher course in her partner's hot spots. The penis is the most significant part of male sexual anatomy. Knowing how to excite the different parts—glans, frenulum, and shaft—will greatly enhance his sexual experience, as will stimulating his testicles, perineum, and anus, all of which are rich in nerve endings. So sit back and take notes—here is the male member demystified once and for all.

The penis

The penis is made up of spongy erectile tissue. This becomes rigid when it is filled with blood, which happens as a response to being aroused.

Despite the slang "boner," a penis has no bone. But it can break (or perhaps a more apt term is "bend") if it hits a hard surface during sex, such as your pubic bone or the headboard of your bed. This can be extremely painful, but usually heals without harm.

Glans and frenulum

The glans is the head of the penis. This highly sensitive tissue has been compared to a woman's clitoris, as both are made out of the same tissue. If the man has not been circumsized, the glans of the unerect penis is covered by the foreskin. Men find stimulation of this area to be highly erotic.

His frenulum can be found on the underside of his penis, and is a small fold of skin where the glans meets the shaft. This is a particularly pleasurable spot on most men, since it is rich in sensitive nerve endings.

Shaft

The shaft is the length of the penis, which extends from the base to the head, and varies from man to man. The average penis is about six inches long. Most men are within the five- to seven-inch range, but variations along this scale are not unusual, and penises of any size can stimulate a woman sexually. Stroking the ridge, which runs the length of the underside of his penis, will usually excite an erection. Run your fingertips along it gently, or pleasure it with long firm licks of your tongue.

One of the most sensitive spots on a man's penis is the frenulum. It is rich in nerve endings and stimulating it yields exquisite sensations.

Foreskin

The foreskin is the flap of skin that covers the glans of an uncircumcized penis. When the penis is erect, the foreskin retracts to just above the glans. Pulling back the foreskin and gently rubbing underneath is very pleasurable.

Many men have had their foreskin removed via circumcision, a controversial practice in some cultures. There is no medical evidence to suggest a clear need for it, but some medical practitioners believe it promotes better genital hygiene.

Urethra

The urethra is located at the opening of the glans. It connects from the bladder to the tip of the penis—this is the opening through which sperm and urine leave the body. Stimulation of the urethra can be very pleasurable for men, some of whom even insert tiny rods into their urethra. Known as "sounding," this is often used in S&M roleplay as a form of power exchange.

Testicles and scrotum

A man's testicles are located below his penis and are covered in a sack of skin known as the scrotum. The testes are the male sex glands and contain his sperm, which are stored in a coiled duct called the epididymis. Sperm are either male or female, and are produced by men from puberty onward. There is no upper limit for men's fertility—unlike women, men can continue to be fertile into their nineties and beyond.

When your partner is aroused almost to the point of orgasm, his sperm is carried from the testicles in two tubes (one from each testicle) called the vas deferens to the two seminal vesicles, located on each side of the bladder. Here the sperm mixes with seminal fluid ready to be discharged during ejaculation.

The testes probably developed outside the male body because sperm fare best in an environment that is cooler than normal body temperature. Men who are looking to father children can promote healthy sperm production with a number of simple lifestyle steps, such as eating a healthy diet, and avoiding alcohol, drugs, and tobacco.

Perineum and anus

The perineum is the area located between a man's genitals and anus. It is filled with many tiny nerve endings, which you can stimulate with your fingers, mouth, or even a vibrator.

Inside his anus is the prostate gland. It is located about two inches in on the belly button side. Some men say it feels like a walnut-like bump. Manual stimulation and pressure on the prostate can feel very orgasmic, and some men love to have this area stimulated with a finger or sex toy. You can access your partner's prostate by inserting your finger or a sex toy into his anus, or by applying deep pressure through his perineum.

Male sexual anatomy

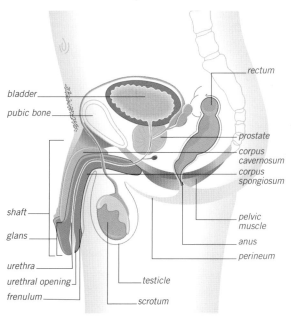

bladder
pubic bone
rectum
prostate
corpus cavernosum
corpus spongiosum
pelvic muscle
anus
perineum
shaft
glans
urethra
urethral opening
frenulum
testicle
scrotum

Connecting with your body

Sexual empowerment begins with high self-esteem and positive body image. When you feel confident about your appearance, size, and shape, you are more likely to want to have sex. Feeling sexy also means you are more likely to try new positions, ideas, or sexual techniques. Whether you are curvaceous, delicate, muscular, thin, or plump, your body type is part of your sexuality. And the sexiest women are those who are comfortable in their skin, confident in their sexuality, and uninhibited in the bedroom.

Understand your sex appeal

Believe it or not, your sex appeal is not about your body shape, weight, height, or breast size. It is all about what you do with your body, and how you show it off. The female body was not designed with the latest fashions, a certain pair of jeans, or a thong in mind. It was designed to attract a mate. And men find all sorts of body shapes attractive—from soft, curving lines to abundant, fleshy bits.

The body in the media

The female body has always been a source of inspiration for artists. From the naked splendor of Rubens' plump beauties to Audrey Hepburn's waiflike frame, the female body—in its many forms—has become part of our identity.

Yet while women with hourglass figures, such as Marilyn Monroe, were once heralded for their sexy, real curves, women today are expected to have the bodies of prepubescent girls. Hips are out, curves are out, and breasts must be appropriately perky and youthful. If you look at pictures of female celebrities in magazines, you will soon notice that our standard of beauty is going through a "skinny" phase.

Taking control of your image

As a result, many women have poor body image or believe their bodies need to be fixed in some way. The signature things that make us who we are—freckles, moles, stretch marks, curves, breast size and shape—are the very things we spend half our time trying to erase.

Connecting with your body is an important part of tuning in to your sex life. If you aren't comfortable with what you see in the mirror, you will no doubt feel uncomfortable being unclothed in front of your partner. Keeping your body under wraps will only serve to lessen your joy in the bedroom, and your partner's, too.

It is possible to learn to love your body, both for the amazing feats it is capable of, and for its pure aesthetic beauty, which it offers to all who are lucky enough to see it in its full glory.

Harmonize your mind and body

Women who enjoy satisfying and exuberant sex lives don't worry about their bodily appearance. They believe their body is sexy and are not inhibited by their cellulite or wrinkles. When your mind takes a more positive attitude toward your body, you also start to realize how sexy you are.

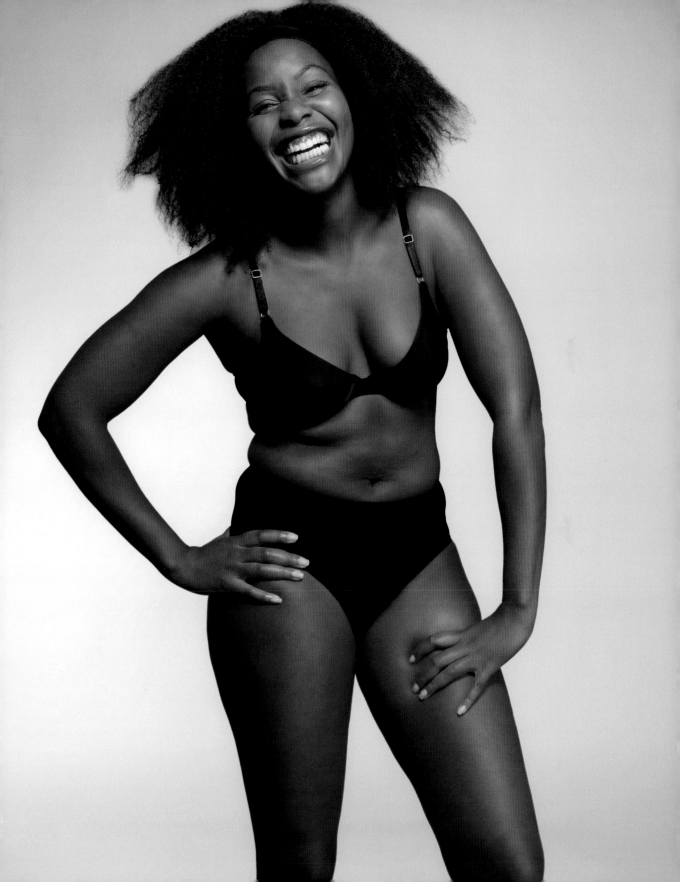

Start by looking at your body and appreciating your positive qualities—it might be your cute feet, heavy breasts, long eyelashes, super-shiny hair, or marvelous curves. Be proud of your body by standing tall and showing off your best parts, whether it's your deep cleavage or nice bum.

Remember that your sex appeal is all of you—the way you walk and talk, your expression, and your body language. Being happy and confident is sexy. Smiling is sexy. What looks good on the catwalk is not what turns your man on between the sheets—it is your own unique shape and feel.

Pass on your positive views about your body to your daughters and granddaughters, and they will grow up in a much more positive environment, which embraces all types of beauty.

Lighten up over weight

The top body concern of most women is their weight. If you feel fat and flabby, you are less likely to want to be uninhibited in the bedroom.

Most women are actually about the right size, but are unhappy with their shape because they compare themselves with women in the media. But those women achieve their—sometimes unhealthily thin—bodies by intensive weight-loss and fitness regimens. Even a fit, healthy woman would be hard-pressed to achieve the body of a young celebrity. When you factor in pregnancy, motherhood, full-time careers, menopause, and aging, you realize what an unattainable goal we set for ourselves. We don't need to please the camera or magazine editors, we just need to feel sexy for ourselves and our partner.

There are many positive actions you can take to feel better about your weight. Keep the scale out of sight. If you weigh yourself more than once a week, you are more likely to struggle with weight and body issues. Instead, note how your clothes fit you—are they tighter or looser?—and use that as a way to gauge weight loss or gain. And avoid diet foods. Anything with the word "diet" in it is best avoided. Instead, simply eat healthily. And buy clothes that flatter your shape rather than worrying about the size on the label.

Remember, many men adore larger women, and usually don't notice if their partner gains or loses a few pounds. As far as they are concerned, more pounds equals more curves. But most men do hate diet talk—hearing you moan about your weight is not conducive to a good sex life.

If you need to lose weight for health reasons, find a diet or healthy-eating program that suits your lifestyle. Consider joining a weight-loss club. The mutual support and encouragement from other women can really improve your chances of losing weight. Enjoy your sex life now, and look forward to a healthier you when you have lost the surplus pounds.

Feel good with exercise

You will reap the rewards of a better sex life if you add exercise to your routine. A cardiovascular workout is a natural mood enhancer, and will make you feel good about the fact that you are taking positive steps to achieving a fitter, firmer, and overall more healthy body—all of which will make you feel better about showing it off.

Your sex appeal is all of you—the way you walk and talk, your expression, and your body language. Being happy and confident is sexy.

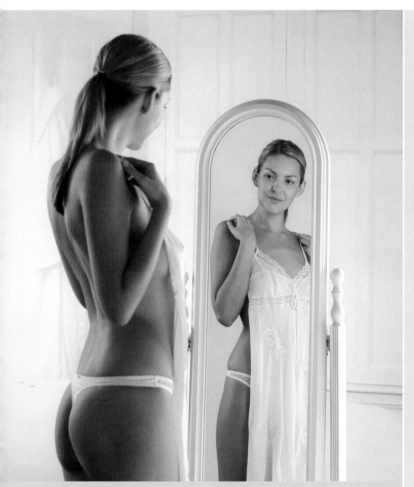

Take a long look at yourself

Connect with your body by treating it with care and indulging your senses. Embrace yourself—focus on your positive aspects. Adapt your wardrobe—make sure your clothes play up your features. Luxuriate—pamper yourself. Look at your whole body, your face, your skin, your shape—you will find that you are a beautiful package.

Embrace

Take some photographs of yourself and your friends enjoying yourselves and put them up around your home. Every time you see pictures in which you look confident and happy, you will instantly feel your mood lift. From this point onward, beware your media influences. If you get a negative body image after reading a particular fashion magazine or watching a TV show, then give it up. This signifies a new beginning—a beginning in which your flaws become your assets, and you accept your body as beautiful.

Adapt

Take an honest look at the clothes in your closet—they say a lot about your body image. Do the colors complement your skin and hair tone? Does the cut make the most of your body shape and size? Edit your wardrobe. If an item isn't getting worn, ask yourself why. Then either give it another try, or donate it to charity. And next time you are out shopping, be sure to buy clothes that highlight your feminine curves and make you feel good about yourself.

Luxuriate

Treat your body to a sensory time out. Fill up the bathtub with warm, bubbly water, light some candles, and turn on your favorite CD. Luxuriate in the water for at least an hour— no phones, obligations, or guilt allowed. As you bathe, run your hands all over your body. Notice how sensual and warm it feels. When you get out of the tub, rub sweet-smelling lotion over yourself. Revel in the sensation of appreciating your body.

Sex files: Learning to love yourself

Poor body image and low self-esteem can have a profoundly negative effect on your love life—if you're feeling unattractive, the last thing you'll want to do is to have sex. Here's how one woman overcame her negative feelings and embraced a reinvigorated sex and personal life.

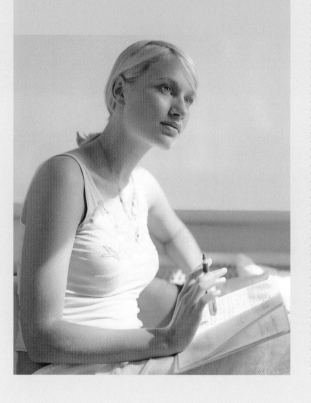

Background

Two years ago Anna, 37, discovered that her husband Jo was having an affair. While they were trying to rebuild their marriage, she found out he was cheating again—with a woman he'd met online. This time Anna asked Jo to leave and she filed for divorce. A year after her divorce was finalized, Anna began dating again. After several months she met a man she was crazy about—Kamal—and now they are settling happily into a relationship. Anna has two children from her marriage to Jo.

The problem

Although Anna felt passionately about Kamal, she didn't enjoy sex and was lukewarm about his sexual advances.

After a hormone test ruled out any underlying physiological reasons for Anna's lack of libido, I spoke at length to her about her feelings and attitudes toward sex. It turned out that, in the past, Anna had really enjoyed sex and was always very adventurous. "I used to feel very confident and daring. Out of all my friends, I was the one to experiment. They used to ask me for sex advice!" Anna's sexually adventurous spirit and healthy libido ended when she discovered her ex-husband's infidelity.

When I told Anna I thought low self-esteem was part of the reason for her lack of interest in sex, she became very emotional. "I've felt so low since Jo cheated on me," she said. "I know Kamal loves me, but I'm waiting for him to find somebody thinner, sexier, or younger than me. I just feel like an overweight single mom—men don't find me attractive or sexy."

Finding solutions

I spoke to Anna and Kamal together. I asked Anna to share her feelings with Kamal in a non-blaming way, and I advised Kamal not to try to "fix" her feelings. When couples encounter self-esteem issues, it's very common for one partner to pooh-pooh the other's feelings. Unfortunately, telling someone that they are wrong to have a negative self-perception doesn't help—self-esteem must be built from within.

To boost Anna's self-esteem I asked her to throw out all her fashion and celebrity magazines (studies show that women experience lower self-esteem after reading them). I also advised her to go to an exercise class and to begin a gratitude journal, in which she would write down one thing she was grateful for every day.

To boost her sexual self-confidence I sent Anna to a sexy lingerie store and asked her to buy at least three sexy garments. Sexy underwear can help to make you feel in control of your sexuality. I also asked Anna to get in tune with her body and her sexual responses by masturbating.

Finally, I asked Anna to put all her ugly, hurtful thoughts toward Jo in a letter. I then told her to burn the letter and let that part of her life go.

What happened?

Anna rebuilt her self-esteem slowly but surely. She joined a Pilates class and made some new friends (bonding with other women can be a crucial part of self-esteem construction). She worked hard at putting her experiences with Jo behind her and she started enjoying sex with Kamal. She said: "When Kamal tells me how much he desires me, I've actually started to believe him—that makes him feel good too."

Regaining confidence
If you have body-image issues that stop you from enjoying sex, try to face them. Make a list of all the things you need to do to feel better about yourself—then do them. And, if possible, avoid the people, activities, or reading material that dent your self-confidence.

Masturbation for women

Masturbation is a natural part of human sexuality, and an important facet of a healthy sex life. Regular orgasms help decrease stress, increase genital blood flow, and promote a better sexual response. You have sexual needs that require satisfying, and masturbation is a reliable path to fulfilment, as well as educating yourself about your body. Masturbation will also help you learn about your sexual response—knowledge that you can use to enhance lovemaking sessions with your partner.

A natural behavior

Contrary to many people's beliefs, masturbation is healthy sexual behavior. However, many women feel uncomfortable about it. For example, they rarely discuss masturbation among themselves or with their partners. But whoever you are, whether you admit it or not, everybody masturbates. In fact, it has been revealed as the most common human sexual activity. And why not? It feels great, it is good for you, and it is the only sexual activity that is 100 percent safe.

What's more, masturbation can relieve sexual tension, and will teach you about your body's responses and how to achieve an orgasm. Those who don't indulge may miss out on achieving maximum pleasure.

Get in the mood

Now that you have had your anatomy lesson, you should be able to find your hot spots—such as the clitoris and G-spot—with the help of a hand mirror or some explorative touching. But locating these hot spots is just the beginning. Getting yourself into a relaxed state of mind, and then knowing how to stimulate yourself, are equally vital parts of the process.

Different strokes

When it comes to masturbation, most women have their preferences. Some enjoy soft, light brushes, while others enjoy hard, fast strokes. Some women like to use their hands or a vibrator, while other women prefer a handheld showerhead or pillow to reach a climax.

In order to discover what you enjoy, make sure you masturbate regularly. Play with different positions and techniques to find out which are the most enjoyable. You will find that self-love can give you some helpful clues for what you will enjoy during sex.

Take your time

A wonderfully relaxing way to enjoy your self-love time is in a bathtub full of warm and bubbly water. To create the right mood, light some candles and put on some relaxing music. Savor the moment and, as you bathe, run your hands over your body, and then between your legs. Get carried away with the sensuality of it all.

Explore and experiment in order to find out what works best for you—and enjoy the intense sensations of your fingers and the warm water against your genitals.

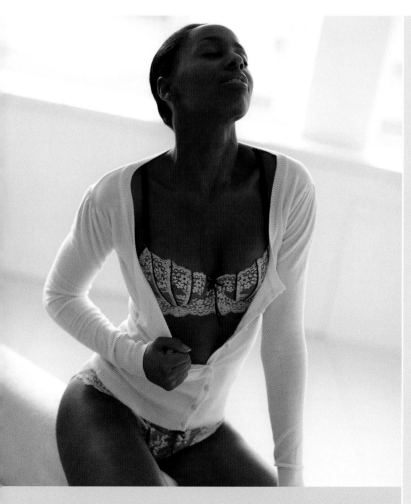

Touch

Zero in on your erogenous zones—breasts, nipples, inner thighs, torso, and stomach. Discover what body part sends chills down your spine. Gently tickle and caress your inner thighs, massage your breasts, and stimulate your nipples. Listen to your body and discover what erotic zones raise your heart rate and get you excited—technically we all have the same hot spots, but we also have our preferences. So take your time and explore every area of your body.

Rub

Try rubbing different parts of your genitals—vulva, vagina, periurethral area, clitoris, and perineum. Experiment with different types of movement—up and down, back and forth, round and round. Even if you masturbate often and have regular orgasms, you can enhance your excitement and intensify the experience by taking your time and trying out different strokes and pressures.

Imagine

If you find it hard to shut out the world and just revel in the pleasures of self-love, close your eyes and bring to mind a sexy image or fantasy. Let your mind run wild and imagine the sensual pleasures of your fantasy in detail—feel the warm sand beneath your naked body, or the muscles in your fantasy-man's arms. Use your imagination to enrich the sensations that your fingers are creating. There aren't any rules you need to stick to, so feel free to create the most vivid fantasies and enjoy satisfying your wildest sexual desires, no matter what they might be.

Loving yourself

Plan time alone for yourself and make sure the environment is relaxing. Don't make an orgasm the goal, or you will become stressed and disappointed if it doesn't happen. Instead focus on feeling sensual and touching your body in ways that feel pleasurable. Whether or not an orgasm occurs, enjoy this special time alone to relax your mind and body.

Masturbation for men

Male masturbation practices have long been the stuff of legend. Men are just less inhibited about sex. Most men accept they have sexual needs and are practiced in satisfying themselves. Your partner probably knows what strokes turn him on, and which produce the best orgasms. In fact, he would probably love to show you all his favorite moves. Self-love doesn't have to be restricted to private moments—it can be an exciting way to teach each other about your bodies and how to turn them on.

No more secrets

Men might be more open about masturbation, but, like women, they learned to masturbate in secret when they were young—they didn't want their mom walking in on them. As a result, their rituals probably began as a private, quiet, and frantic activity—something to be indulged in when they could be left alone without interruption.

In later life, men may still view masturbation as something to be done as quickly and quietly as possible, and behind a locked door. This means they don't reap the full pleasure benefits, and they are actually training their bodies to reach ejaculation as quickly as possible.

Men can break away from this rushed state of mind by setting aside some time when they know they won't be disturbed. Encourage your man to enjoy his self-love time by passing on these tips.

Make it smooth

When it comes to male masturbation, lubrication is important. Genital skin is delicate and prone to dryness and abrasion. After repeated strokes, masturbation can become painful if the penis is not fully lubricated. Lotion or baby oil can be effective, and a warming-type lubricant can feel very erotic. Some lubricants also have a numbing action, for men wanting to extend and enhance their sexual performance.

A self-love session

Like women, a man should find a place to masturbate where he feels comfortable and relaxed. Many men find that masturbating in the shower can be especially satisfying, as the warm sensation of the water provides added stimulation and excitement to their self-love session.

Talking about masturbation will open the door to other sexual discussions. You might reveal your favorite fantasies and discover his.

Getting naked is a good way to start—he will then find it helpful to spend five minutes or so breathing deeply and just letting his mind relax. It is important that a man enjoy this time with himself and get pleasure from it— he might also learn something about his sexual response.

Men react to visual stimulation, so he might want to use an erotic magazine or movie, or to imagine a favorite fantasy to become aroused.

Once he's getting in the mood, he can touch his body lightly all over, then use stronger, firmer strokes on his chest, thighs, and buttocks. Then, when he is feeling fully aroused, he can move on to stroking and caressing his genitals.

There are also many sex toys designed to enhance male masturbation and they can add novelty to his routine in the bath or bedroom. Once he climaxes, there's no need to rush and finish the session. Instead, he should try to spend a few minutes relaxing and enjoying the sense of release and peace.

Build stamina, create intimacy

Masturbating is a pleasurable solo pursuit for a man, but it also has the benefit of improving the sex you have with him. This is because regular self-love sessions build up his stamina and result in more powerful and prolonged orgasms. And being open with your partner about your self-love practices can bring you closer together.

If you and your partner have never spoken about your sexual needs or preferences, then talking about masturbation will open the door to other sexual discussions. These might include revealing your favorite fantasies and discovering his. You may also discover how often you both want sex—and which positions you both enjoy most. Being open with each other about these matters will naturally enhance your intimacy and understanding of each other. In this way, and others, masturbation can do wonders for both of your arousal levels and sex drives.

Mutual masturbation

Many people fantasize about watching their lover masturbate and it can be a very erotic experience. Start by touching yourself, then watch your partner's touches. Don't rush to reach a mutual orgasm—watching each other climax in turn can be a freeing experience. It can also be the best prologue to manual sex. Once you've put on a show for your partner, he'll know all the right touches to use when it's his turn to play.

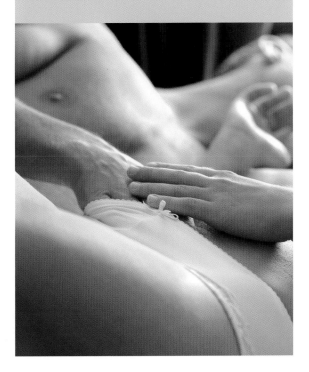

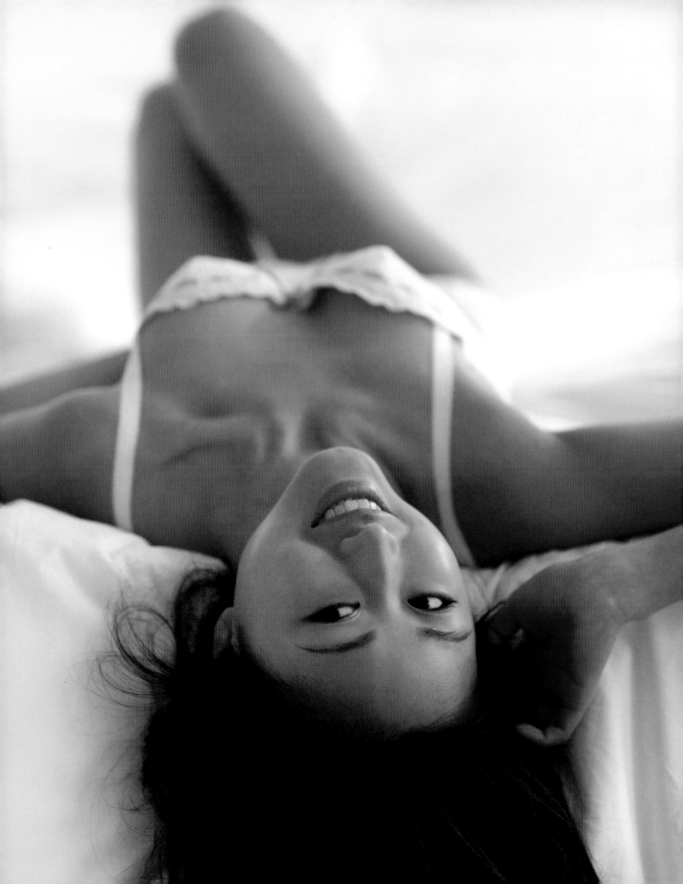

Know your mind

What are your thoughts about sex? It is important to reflect on this, because the images and words that come into your mind when you are having sex can affect your sexual response and your enjoyment. Making sure your mind is on board is an important part of having a good sex life—after all, your brain is your biggest sex organ. Your mind and your emotional health are intimately tied to your libido. So direct your thoughts to enhancing your self-esteem, and concentrate on releasing your inner seductress to get the most out of your relationship.

Perspectives on sex

Women are beautiful, multifaceted, sexual creatures, designed to enjoy lovemaking. Evolution made us that way for good reason—we play an important role in keeping the human race going. However, inadequate early teaching or experiences can make it difficult for some women to enjoy sex as a natural and pleasurable act. It is impossible to realize your potential if you are harboring negative thoughts about your sexuality. In fact, it does us all good now and again to examine our views on sex.

The seeds of sexual beliefs

From your first chaste kiss on the playground to the first time you made love, your initiation into the world of sex has the power to color your sexual future. Decades may have passed, but these potent memories are probably still with you. And although negative experiences might not prevent you from engaging in sex altogether, they might make you less orgasmic during sex, or less willing to try new positions or activities.

The media, with their conflicting images of female sexuality, also has a significant impact on our beliefs. On the one hand, we are shown that women should be sexy, orgasmic, and free-spirited. But on the other hand, sexual naivety is shown to be desirable. The truth is that women can't accomplish sexual freedom if they are not free to experiment with different partners and to enjoy sex without fear of being labeled.

Set your own agenda

Sex is a natural and healthy part of being human, though it does attract labels—from ourselves and from others. But trying a new sex position or act does not make a woman a slut. You can play the whore in the bedroom, or act naive. It is okay to beg for sex and it is perfectly acceptable to say "no." These are simply different sexual behaviors. They do not define you as a person—they are part of a normal sexual repertoire.

Once you think about your sexual beliefs you will be better able to accept your own sexuality, and set your standards. Maybe you don't believe in one-night stands, or that sex should be kept to committed relationships. It helps to define your sexuality before communicating it to potential partners. As long as you aren't hurting anyone and your sex life is emotionally and physically healthy, it is yours to explore, adore, and enjoy.

Record your thoughts

If you are struggling to let go of negative sexual encounters or want to uncover your views on sex, try keeping a journal. Make a list of goals, such as "I want to be more uninhibited." Then list the things that are preventing you from reaching your goals, such as "I need to feel comfortable naked." Once you realize what action you need to take, you can address them alone or with your partner.

If you still find yourself struggling to enjoy sex, a sex therapist can help you work through your feelings about your sexuality.

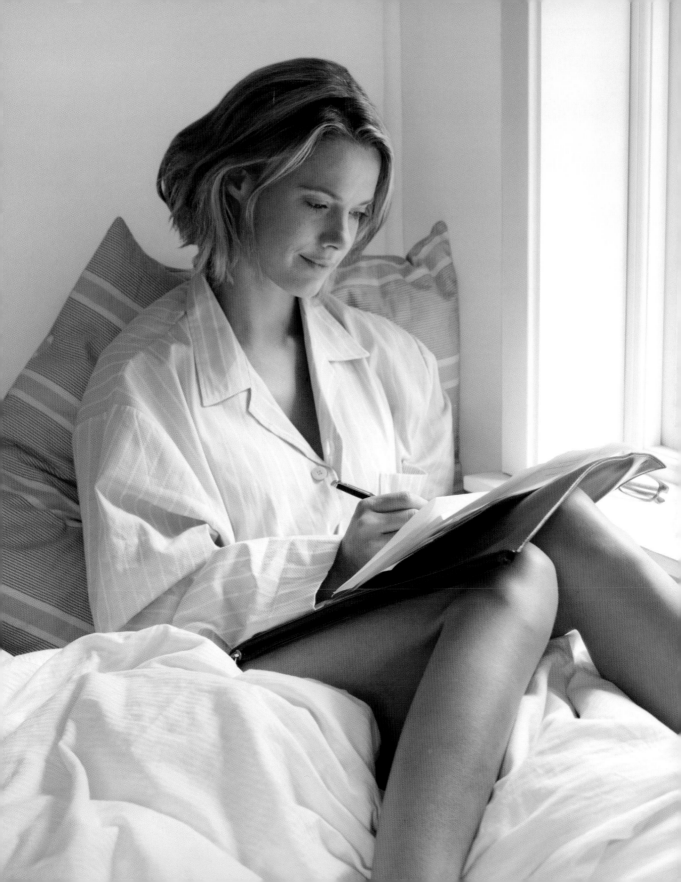

Self-esteem and your sex life

A woman with good self-esteem is confident and uninhibited in the bedroom. Her outlook on life is positive and she is motivated to attain a happy and fulfilling sex life. Why? Because if you feel good about yourself, you are more likely to be adventurous and try new things. If you are confident, you appreciate yourself as a woman and make your sexual needs a priority. And if you feel fantastic and sexually satisfied in body and mind, you walk down the street with a smile and a sway in your hips.

Identify the obstacles to self-esteem
Feeling unattractive, unappreciated, stressed, and anxious can lead to negative self-esteem. Ill health, aging, fertility problems, and even family disagreements can also leave you feeling uncertain and unhappy. On the other hand, if you are contented, fulfilled, and relaxed you are more likely to find sexual satisfaction.

Think and act yourself happy
Self-esteem and happiness depend on self-acceptance. Look in the mirror every day, and repeat this mantra until it becomes part of your being: "I am in charge of my actions. I control my own happiness. I accept and love myself." Saying these words on a regular basis will boost your self-esteem and put you on a path that acknowledges you are worthy of self-respect and love.

Combat negative feelings about yourself by embracing your potential. Take up a sport, such as jogging, volleyball, tennis, or even walking. Push yourself—you might be surprised at just how strong you are. And try it with your partner: you will get an endorphin rush from working out together, which is bound to create sexual sparks later on in the bedroom.

Create your personal space
Spend time alone. Browse in a bookstore, or just sit and watch the world go by. This allows you to free your mind and think about your life. Rest and relaxation are vital to improving your state of mind, and let you review your sexual relationship.

There are many ways to create happiness for yourself. Spend time on activities that replenish your spirit, whether it is talking with friends,

Break out of the ordinary and create some excitement. Try a new position, buy a sexy perfume, or wear barely-there underwear.

having dinner with your children, or pursuing a hobby. Alternatively, devote yourself to a good cause, whether it's volunteering at a local charity or pitching in with a community service project. Helping those in need will make you feel better about yourself. And feeling better about yourself will help you tune into your sensuality.

Make a show of your sexuality

Take your partner somewhere new, such as a trendy restaurant or a salsa class. Breaking out of the ordinary could help you both get out of a rut, and create some excitement and positive energy.

This extends to the bedroom. Try a new position, buy a sexy perfume, or wear barely-there underwear. You will find that if you do things that make you feel pleased with yourself, you will enjoy an immediate boost in self-esteem.

Confront your body-image fears and excite your partner by making love with the lights on. He finds you attractive—that is why he is having sex with you. Let him see your body in all its beautiful (and, yes, imperfect) glory. He wants to see every curve and freckle, and the pleasure on your face when you reach orgasm. His approval will boost your self-esteem and encourage you to be even more adventurous next time.

Secure your path to satisfaction

Self-esteem and a great sex life aren't by-products of looking good. Whether you want to start your own company, become a mother, or receive a promotion at work, working hard to accomplish your ambitions creates positive self-esteem. That confidence in turn enhances every area of your life, including sex.

On your journey of self-discovery, you might find it helpful to have a mentor or heroine—a family member, a woman you admire, or a fictional character. Think of her whenever you feel weak on your journey. And remember: making your dreams come true is the best mood enhancer out there.

Find your super-boost

Set yourself a challenge that forces you out of your comfort zone. Take up dancing, run a marathon, join a theater group. It can be anything, even putting on a sexy display for your partner, as long as you discover or express something new about yourself. This will boost your self-confidence and inspire further feats. It will also help you find the sensual woman within, who knows how to please herself and her partner.

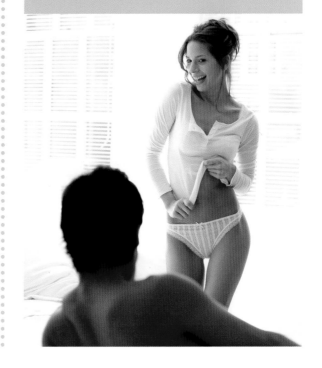

Self-esteem and your partner's sex life

Women aren't the only ones who are at the mercy of poor self-esteem. Men are just as likely to suffer a lack of confidence in their own abilities, but they tend not to talk about it. All sorts of events and emotions will contribute to low self-esteem, but their power can be defused with some positive thinking and emotional boosts. A man with high self-esteem is confident in his skills as a lover and provider, which results in a healthy emotional and sexual relationship with his partner.

The obstacles to his self-esteem

The main obstacles to a man attaining high self-esteem tend to be connected with his traditional, and still relevant, social role of provider. Failure to achieve his goals, being dominated by a partner, poor fertility or sexual problems, financial worries, ill health, and feeling unattractive and unfit can all lead to poor self-esteem.

Losing his job or being passed over for promotion will also deeply affect his feelings of self-worth and may have a negative impact on your sex life until they are resolved. These are difficult challenges for any couple to face.

Pledge your support

Not suprisingly, men experience the same deleterious effects of low self-esteem that women do—low energy, low motivation, and low sex drive.

What's more, if his self-esteem has taken a beating, it is easy to damage it further by being critical or anxious.

Help him find ways to rebuild his confidence. Support him and give him ideas to resolve his work problems, if he asks. Maintaining some form of intimacy is very important during these times.

Lift his confidence

If you want to enjoy a healthy sex life, it is vital your man knows you find him attractive. Write yourself a mental note to compliment your partner every day. Tell him he is looking handsome, heathier, or more toned. Your emotional boosts will make him feel happier and consequently improve his sex drive. And if he is feeling good about himself, he is more likely to reflect the positive ego boosts back to the source—you.

Compliment his sexual prowess. Many men associate manhood with being a knockout in bed, so praise him on his staying power.

It is also important to compliment his sexual prowess. Many men associate manhood with being a knockout in bed, so praise him on his staying power or genital appearance. Keep your compliments specific and genuine, such as "I love how tender you are when we make love," or "I love how you always hit the right spot."

Focus on the good things

Accentuate the positive in your relationship and ignore the negative. In other words, thanking your partner for his compliment will remind him to do it more often. Knowing that you appreciate his effort goes a long way to making him feel good about your relationship and sex life.

The more you build up this feeling of positivity, the more it becomes a reality—helping to squeeze out the negative in the process.

Share your success

If your man's self-esteem is low, you can boost it by spending time together doing activities that give you shared goals—such as hiking or bike riding. The exercise will also improve his mental outlook and lead to good bedroom vibes.

Notice his achievements. Men don't always toot their own horn when they have had a good day at work. Ask for the details and applaud his efforts. This will boost his ego and encourage him to continue being successful. If he feels happy and appreciated, he is more likely to want to celebrate with you in bed.

Give him time

Just as your partner doesn't always fill you in when he's had a good day, he might also be inclined to hide his emotions about a bad one. Don't push him for details, but offer your support by letting him know that you're there for him. Be patient, since he might take a little while to come out of his shell. While you are waiting, a spot of quiet time can be therapeutic for both of you.

Private playtime

If you want to help de-stress your lover, invite him to the bedroom for some adult playtime. Any sexual activity is a great way to unwind together—and your invitation will boost his self-esteem. Get yourselves in the mood with some simple silliness. Play around taking pictures of your lover, challenge him to a pillow fight, or tell each other jokes and funny stories while lying naked in bed.

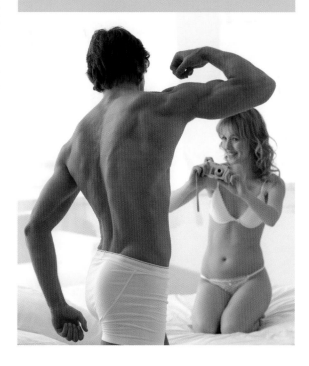

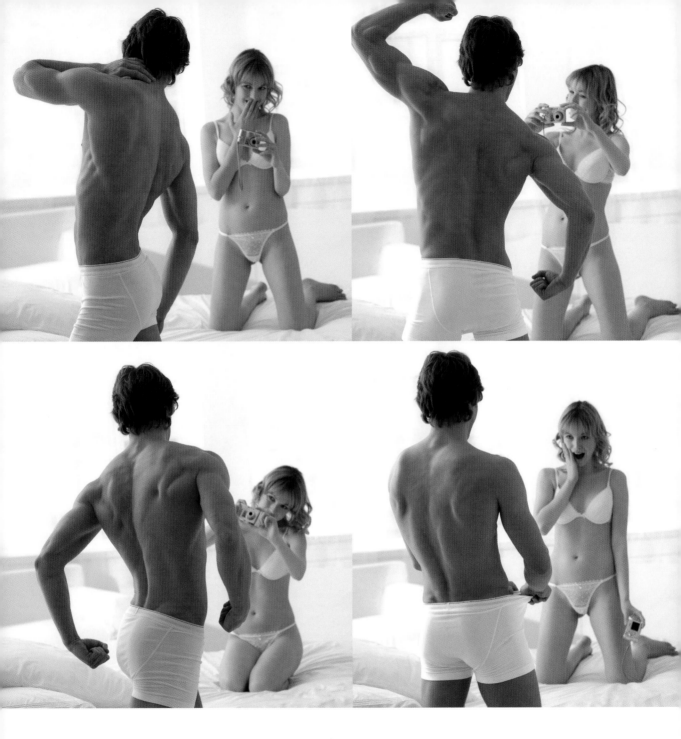

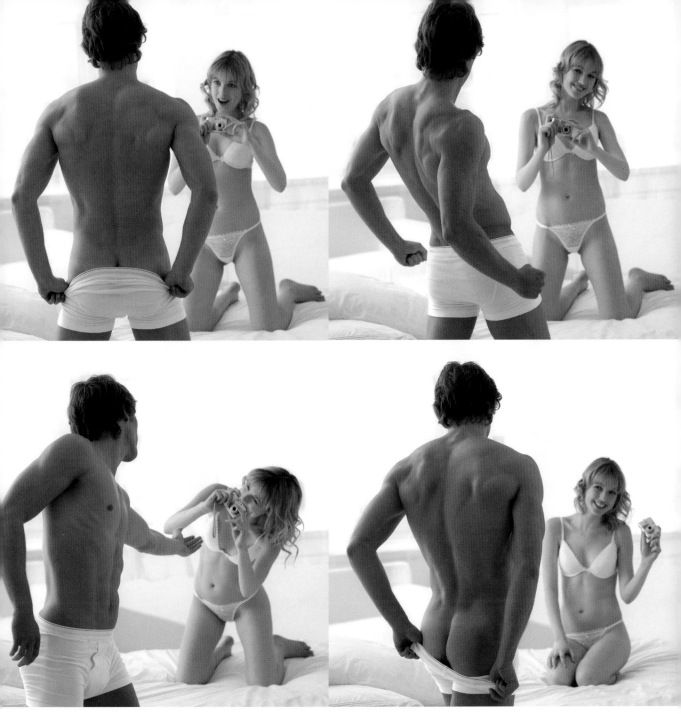

Demand a private viewing

▲ Pay your partner the ultimate compliment and ask him to perform a strip show for the camera. Make it fun, admire his body, and offer thoughtful compliments. When he feels confident in his body, he is more likely to reward you with some esteem-boosting activity between the sheets.

Sex drive

A person's libido, otherwise known as sexual desire, is often simply defined as their interest in sex. This interest in sex is governed by a number of different factors, such as your physiological urges, emotional impulses, and psychological needs. A healthy libido is also dependent on our other basic needs being met, which usually means that food, sleep, and rest come first. But once they are satisfied, the mood for emotional and physical intimacy comes on strong.

The power of the libido

A woman with a strong libido has satisfied all her basic needs so she is able to focus on the more pleasurable parts of life, such as sex and her relationships. Libido also affects more than your sex life—it is a powerful mood enhancer and will enable you to embrace other aspects of your life, including your emotional and creative energy.

Not in the mood

Even a strong libido has off days. Normally you'd be ready to rip off your partner's shirt, but there are times—if you've had a bad day, for instance, or if you are tired and stressed—when you might just not be in the mood for sex.

Since libido is affected by so many different factors, it can be hard to pinpoint the culprit behind a low libido. Finding it is the first step to revitalizing your sex drive. There is generally a combination of factors to blame—medical problems, stress, hormonal disturbances, poor health, relationship disturbances, medications, low self-esteem, and negative sexual experiences all play a role in decreased or diminishing sex drive.

Maintaining a strong libido

A common myth is that our sex drive is lost as we age. While it is true that men and women sometimes both experience dwindling libido as they age, strong libido really has no age limit.

While you can't control getting older, you can control the factors that affect your libido. Watch your stress levels, eat well, get plenty of sleep, exercise, and be wary of alcohol and prescription drugs. Do this and your mind will remain free to enjoy sex, and its physical and emotional benefits.

Libido affects more than your sex life. It is a powerful mood enhancer and will enable you to embrace other aspects of your life.

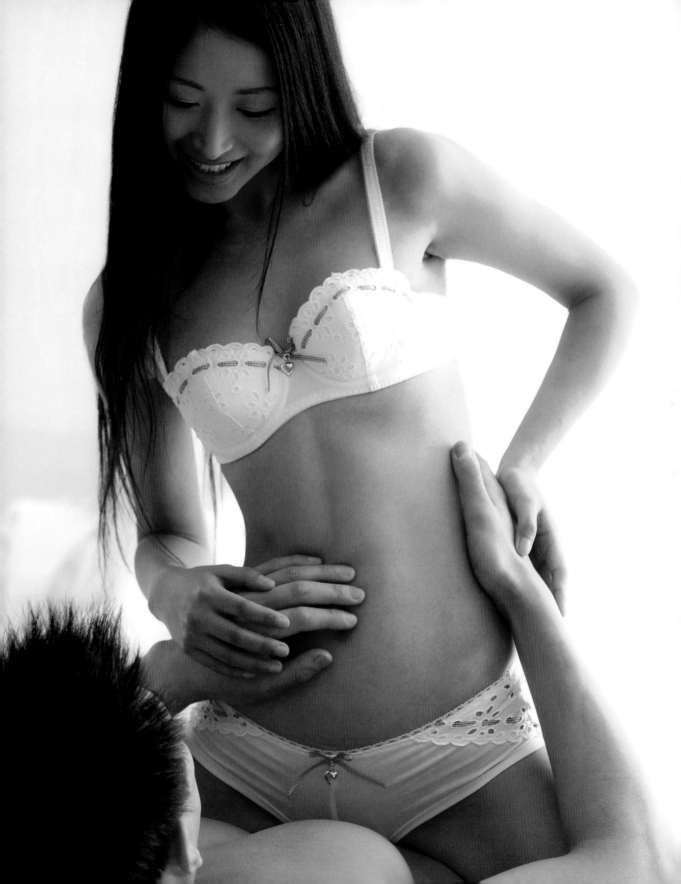

Your sex drive

Your libido is unique to you and is the basis for your sexual enjoyment and interest. How often you have sex is not as important as having a regular and fulfilling sex life. Regular sex promotes good circulation, which increases sexual desire, but the reverse is also true—if you don't have sex or masturbate regularly then your desire and enjoyment will decrease. To enhance your libido, respond to your physical urge to have sex, and be adventurous in your lovemaking.

The role of libido

A healthy libido is at the heart of your sex life. It is a fundamental aspect of your womanhood and your sense of self-fulfilment, and will greatly enhance the intimacy you enjoy with your partner.

But your libido is not constant. It is affected by numerous factors, such as your health, the state of your relationship, and your overall view of life. If you experience a loss of libido over a significant period of time, don't ignore it, as it may be a sign of a deeper physical or emotional problem.

Hormonal obstacles

From the menstrual cycle to pregnancy to menopause, our hormones play a vital role in dictating our fluctuating sexual desire.

However, a common cause of low libido is medication. Hormonal contraceptives (such as pills, patches, and shots) increase your body's production of sex hormone-binding globulin (SHBG), a protein that binds to testosterone. This makes it unavailable to do its work triggering sexual desire and arousal.

Antidepressants, cancer-fighting medication, antihistamines, antihypertensives, sedatives, and ulcer medications can also affect your sex drive.

Ask your doctor about alternative contraceptives and medications, which might have a decreased incidence of sexual side effects.

Lifestyle obstacles

Poor eating habits, a lack of exercise, and other lifestyle choices can negatively affect your libido as well. You need good health and plenty of energy in order to enjoy sex to the fullest.

Alcohol and tobacco give you a temporary high but are not conducive to your long-term well-being or your sex drive. Surviving on a few hours' sleep every night will leave you feeling moody and irritable. Try to get at least seven hours of sleep a night. If this isn't possible, take naps and spend a couple of nights every week catching up on your rest. It might make a big difference to your libido.

Staying on top of stress

Feeling anxious and rushed leads to a build-up of cortisol, which inhibits testosterone and affects your sexual interest. To de-stress, practice relaxation techniques such as meditation and deep breathing throughout the day to help control anxiety. Ultimately, if you take care of your body, your mind will take care of your libido.

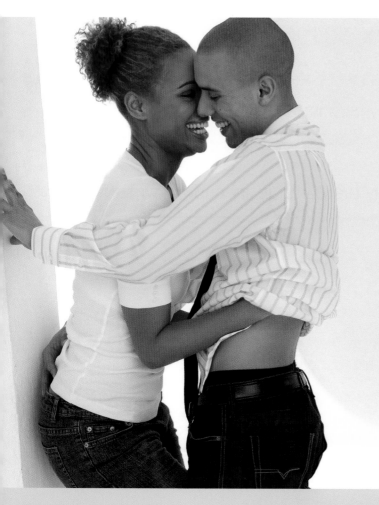

Boosting libido

Your libido is linked to your lifestyle, so if your hormones are out of whack, or you aren't getting regular exercise or eating properly, your libido will suffer. Get these right and you may find that just-got-home kiss with your partner develops into something sexier—and nothing creates a stronger sexual appetite than great sex itself.

Visit your doctor

Menopause and hysterectomy can result in low testosterone levels. The decrease of this hormone can lead to a lower libido. Some women benefit from treatments such as testosterone replacement and hormone therapy. Additionally, sexual problems— such as difficulty reaching orgasm, vaginal dryness, and less-than-intense orgasms— can add to low libido, since sex becomes frustrating or simply unenjoyable. See your doctor promptly to discuss your symptoms and treatment options.

Get active

Keep your health and your libido on track by getting some exercise every day, even if it is just a 20-minute walk or getting off the bus a couple of stops earlier. Endorphins released during physical exercise help to counteract cortisol, which causes your body to hold on to fat. You could also try yoga or abdominal and pelvic exercises, which will help tone your body and increase the strength of your pelvic floor muscles.

Eat wisely

Fried, fatty, and sugary foods not only cause us to gain weight, they also increase insulin levels in our bodies. This can lead to a decrease in the hormones—such as testosterone—that prime our bodies for sex. A balanced diet, which consists of healthy fats and small meals throughout the day, is best for great sex. You can also incorporate a few aphrodisiacs, such as dark chocolate, avocados, oysters, and spicy foods (jalapenos, for example).

Your partner's sex drive

Male libido is often misunderstood. We are socialized to believe that men are ravenous, lustful creatures who have sex on their brains every minute of the day. However, contrary to popular belief, male libido is not based on unmitigated, animal-like lust. It is subject to dips and variations, and is affected by numerous lifestyle and physical factors, just like female libido. Men are as emotionally tied to sex as women are, and most have a need for an emotional bond based on mutual respect and passion.

Understanding male libido

A healthy and active libido is as integral to a satisfying sex life for a man as it is for a woman. Lifestyle factors such as stress, sleep, nutrition, and exercise affect his sex drive as they do yours. His libido is also a direct result of the emotional bond between you, so taking care of your sex life will reflect positively on other aspects of his life, including his career, relationship, and self-esteem.

Emotional obstacles

If you and your partner are having relationship woes, don't be surprised if the tension transfers to the bedroom. We may think men are superheroes who don't cry, but they, too, are affected by perceived slights and relationship difficulties.

Don't ignore conflicts at home, which can lead to feelings of low self-esteem or inadequacy that inevitably affect his—and your—libido. If you strive to resolve emotional difficulties quickly, your sex life and relationship will benefit.

Lifestyle obstacles

Male libido, like female libido, is also subject to the effects of stress. Not surprisingly, too much stress makes a man feel run down and uninterested in sex. Quite often, stress also causes men to sleep less and to eat fatty, libido-killing foods, which may lead to weight gain and a diminished sex drive.

Medication can affect a man's sex drive, just as it affects a woman's. Sedatives, antidepressants, antihistamines, antihypertensives, and cancer-fighting medication can all have an effect. Fortunately, there are prescriptions available that won't have as much of an impact on his libido.

Libido should not have to be sacrificed for good health—the two should go hand-in-hand.

Supplements and herbal remedies

Another way for your partner to keep his libido on track is with supplements and herbal remedies.

Zinc is beneficial to his fertility, and L-arginine is said to increase blood flow to the genital region, which might help to improve his erectile ability. Epimedium (nicknamed "horny goat weed") can help regulate cortisol levels and boost libido in men and women alike. Gingko can help increase blood flow, which helps erectile difficulties, while ginseng enhances stamina and well-being.

Before beginning any herbal regimen, your partner should consult his doctor.

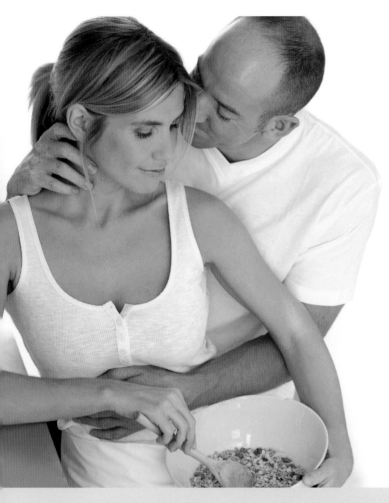

Maintain intimacy

If your partner is suffering from a period of serious stress or lack of sleep, your sex life may suffer as a consequence. If you put pressure on him to perform sexually, or worry him about your poor sex life, you will only serve to decrease his libido further. Help him through his bad times by maintaining intimacy—cuddling, kissing, and touching. Help him find positive resolutions to his problems. His libido will pick up given time, but you can help him recover it by being his positive other half.

Exercise together

Start a new health regimen with your partner by joining a gym and changing your diet. Regular exercise and the right foods, along with your joint understanding and support, might be just what you need to get your sex life back on track. Use the gym as a space to relax between home and work—a neutral place where you can enjoy each other's company and a shared goal to get in shape.

Reduce stress

Negative events can make men feel bad about their bodies. This onslaught of negative feelings can often lead to him suffering from low energy, low motivation, and low sex drive. Try to find a way to help him reduce his stress levels and to attain a calmer attitude. Meditation helps quiet the mind, while life-enhancing exercise such as yoga or tai chi can be very effective. If the stress is ongoing, you may need to make some hard lifestyle choices, such as changing careers or cutting commitments.

Intimate relaxation

You don't have to be in bed to enhance your emotional connection. You can be at the gym, at the movies, in a restaurant. Spend time together at home, being close and intimate. Often, it is when you are both relaxed that he is most interested in sex. These are the times when he can connect with you, and that connection will strengthen his libido.

Mismatched libido

Balancing different sexual needs can be tricky. Your partner may be sexually aroused in the morning, while you prefer nighttime sex. You might crave sex at least once a week, while he seems comfortable forgoing it for a couple of weeks at a time. And while a glimpse of sexy lingerie can get him in the mood, the hunkiest male model couldn't get the same response from you. Every individual is different, but it is possible for a couple with mismatched libidos to a have a good sex life.

Recognize your needs

It is rare to find a couple who have the exact same libido and sexual interest. But this is what makes sex interesting—every person has his or her own sexual needs and sparks, and by discovering each other's needs, we can discover a new sexual side of ourselves.

Create closer bonds

Sex and intimacy go hand-in-hand for men and women. When you don't feel bonded to your partner, you are less likely to want to have sex. And if he senses this lack of interest on your part, you might find his sexual desire also plummets. Take time out each week to connect with your partner on an intimate, nonsexual level—such as cuddling, talking, and simply interacting—and you will find your connection in the bedroom heats up as a result.

Talk about it

One of the most common quarrels couples have is over the amount of sex they are having, or not having. You can manage mismatched libidos in a way that takes your needs and his needs into account—by sharing your sexual wants and desires out loud. This open and honest communication will bring you closer together and help you achieve a deeper and more lasting emotional connection.

What time of day does your partner enjoy having sex? How often does he want sex? Let him know your favorite time and preferred frequency, too. You will find that most of your differences can be addressed with small compromises.

For example, if your partner enjoys early-morning sex, you could agree to morning lovemaking sessions on weekends and holidays but not work days. If you would like to have sex three or four times a week, but he is happy with just once, encourage him by asking what new positions or techniques he would like to try.

Set guidelines for sex

Making bedroom rules might not seem conducive to enhancing your sexual bond, but if external factors are damaging your sex life then you need rules to protect it. These might include installing a lock on the bedroom door to prevent your children from interrupting you, not arguing in the bedroom, and insisting that distractions such as the ironing basket or cell phones are left outside.

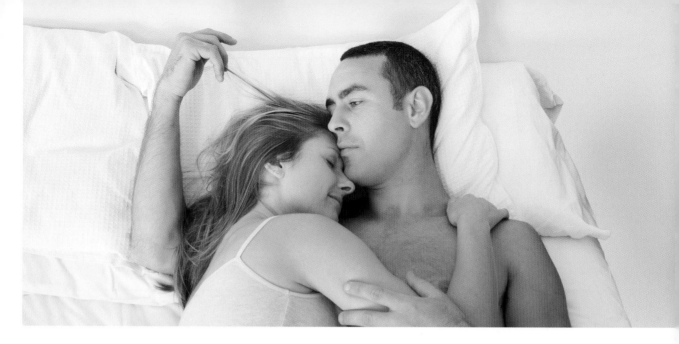

For time-starved couples, a way to protect your sex life is to schedule it. By marking a sex date on the calendar, you and your partner are more likely to follow through. Scheduled sex won't necessarily be romantic, but it is better than no sex at all. It might even be something you look forward to.

Not tonight, darling

If one of you isn't in the mood, you shouldn't feel obligated to have sex. Don't close the door on it entirely—you might find that once the sensual stroking begins, the mood will settle on you or your partner. But pressure to have sex creates hostility and resentment, and a lack of spontaneity and enjoyment. Sex should never feel forced.

You may worry that your libido and your partner's are so severely mismatched that it might ultimately lead to an irreconcilable breakdown in your relationship.

This situation is quite rare since most couples are willing to make the effort to achieve a mutually satisfying sex life. The most important part in managing your different libidos is for both of you to recognize that your sex life is important and valuable, and to commit to working through your sexual issues together.

How therapy can help

If your partner's libido is lower than yours, you need to realize that there is little you can do to change this. Often, the issue behind mismatched libidos is unclear or multi-dimensional. A relationship or sex therapist can help you identify what is causing issues in the bedroom and help you to resolve your differences. Whatever you do, don't dismiss your concerns. When one or both of you aren't having your sexual needs met, it can damage your relationship.

Sex files: Understanding a libido dip

Life events or problems with money can have an impact on your sex drive—this happens to all couples. However, it's possible to create problems and misunderstandings if you don't discuss what is happening. Here's how one couple rescued their relationship from miscommunication.

Background
Kelly, 60, and Luke, 57, have been married for 30 years. They met at school and have two teenage children. Luke runs his own business, which has been failing in recent years. This, coupled with the fact that Kelly doesn't work, means that there is considerable financial strain on the family.

The problem
Despite repeated efforts to seduce him, Kelly felt that Luke no longer wanted sex with her. "He used to be so turned on by me. Just the sight of me getting out of the shower used to give him an erection. Now he doesn't notice me." Her main concern was that Luke was having an affair.

In an individual session with Luke, I asked him about his sex drive. He said he didn't feel like sex because he was so stressed about his debts. He also felt he was failing as a provider and his kids didn't need him anymore. When I explained to Luke that Kelly associated his lack of interest with an affair, he said, "I can't believe she thinks that. It's not like she makes moves on me and I turn her down!"

Finding solutions
My first step was to get Kelly and Luke talking so they could resolve some fairly simple misunderstandings. After explaining to Kelly the reasons for his

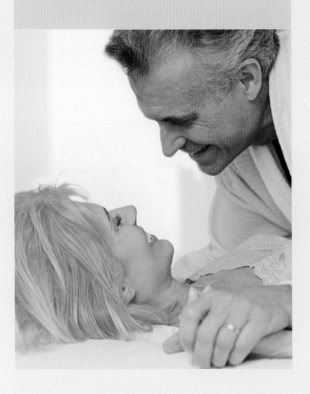

lack of interest in sex, Luke confessed that he couldn't remember when he'd turned down her many advances. Kelly reminded him of a time when she suggested they go to bed early and he chose to stay up and balance the checkbook. Laughing, Luke said, "That was an advance?! I don't notice stuff like that—you have to be more direct."

I agreed with Luke—Kelly did need to be more direct, but so did he. I suggested to Luke that he share his anxieties with Kelly rather than bottling them up. I challenged him to respond to Kelly's questions with at least three different adjectives. So, for example, if Kelly asked, "How was your day?" instead of simply responding "Fine," Luke would have to think of three appropriate words, such as "stressful," "hectic," and "nerve-racking." This would open up Luke's emotions to Kelly so she wouldn't be in the dark about the source of his behavior or moods. I also asked Luke to pay more attention to Kelly in the form of compliments, emails or texts during the day, and kisses and cuddling upon returning home.

Kelly's homework was to initiate sex with Luke at least two times before their next visit to me. I suggested she should send him an x-rated email at work, so he could anticipate seeing her for the rest of the day. Little steps like this can be empowering for women who are shy about making sexual requests. And, since Kelly's sexual advances hadn't been getting through to Luke, I asked her to tune in to the things he considered sexual cues. This included wearing sexy lingerie and playfully touching and teasing Luke.

What happened
Kelly and Luke really enjoyed doing the exercises and said they had become closer than they had been in years. Luke got more sensitive to Kelly's sexual cues and she, in turn, became more overt. And Luke said, "Now, instead of avoiding sex I've started treating it as a way to relax."

Check in with each other
Long-term couples can't expect their libido to be constant. If you notice your partner seems less interested in sex than usual, gently ask them about it. There's no replacement for direct communication, even in the oldest and most familiar of relationships.

Releasing your inner vixen

Every woman has an inner vixen. Who is she? She is the no-holds-barred, carefree, confident, brave, and sexual woman who lives inside all of us. She believes in the power of pleasure, high heels, and red lipstick. She can make an old T-shirt and messy hair look sexy. Men are in awe of her and women envy her—and that woman is you. Perhaps you haven't seen your inner vixen since high school or your last pregnancy. But even if that is the case, she is ready and waiting for you to unleash her once again.

Rediscovering your sex appeal

Underneath the routine and rush of life—and whatever your body-image issues—there is a sexy, seductive, happy, and powerful woman inside of you.

Your inner vixen doesn't necessarily have a perfect body—she is there to encapsulate your seductive potential, and to push you to come up with new ways of displaying it.

But how do you get back in touch with your inner vixen, or discover her for the first time?

Make your surroundings sensual

Your environment, especially the bedroom, should help you channel the carefree, sexy woman inside of you—but this can't happen if you're surrounded by dirty laundry, work documents, and baby bottles.

Clear the clutter: keep office-related items such as your laptop out of the bedroom, along with any childcare paraphernalia. Alternatively, keep a lidded basket or box where you can store any non-bedroom items before you go to bed.

Replace old sheets with more luxurious items in sensual colors or patterns—every time you sink into them, you will feel glamorous and relaxed.

Remove any family pictures hanging on the wall—looking up at an old photo of your parents won't put you in a sexy mood. Install a dimmer on the bedroom light, or use candles when possible. Romantic music and aromatherapy can also help your room feel more inviting and sensual.

Try something new

Our sexy selves often go into hiding because we are too shy or self-conscious to give our sexuality free rein. You may feel you lack the confidence to wear sexy lingerie or to initiate sex with your partner. To bring your vixen back to the surface, you have to leave your comfort zone. Challenge yourself: try a bold new move in the bedroom, such as dirty talk, fantasy role-play, or a new design on your pubic hair. Embrace—and flaunt—the fact that you are sexy.

Seductiveness is in the mind, not the body. It is about feeling open, adventurous, and confident. If you don't feel confident, fake it until you do. Sexiness is the one thing that is okay to fake—and it's guaranteed to help you access your inner vixen. So let down your guard, put your fears aside, and break out your most daring pair of heels—then let your vixen take the lead.

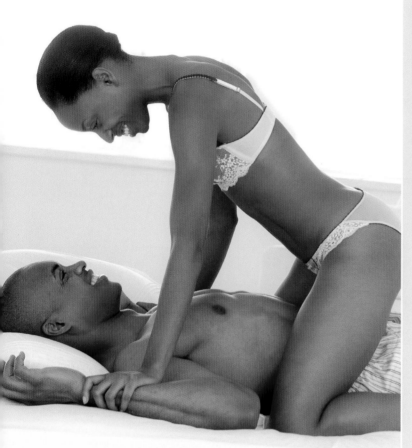

Play the flirt

A little flirty smile at your doorman or waiter is harmless, and it boosts your confidence throughout the day. And just because you have been with your partner for a couple of months, years, or more, it doesn't mean you can't flirt with each other—wink at him across the dinner table, send him an X-rated email, and be vocal about your pleasure in the bedroom. Caress his bottom as you pass in the hall, show him a little thigh, or a lot of cleavage. He will love the new, daring you, and your obvious attraction to him will boost his self-confidence, too.

Seduce him

The next time your partner is having a tough week at work, surprise him with a sexy pampering gift. Run him a hot bubble bath when he gets home and then climb in beside him. Scrub his body, wash his hair, then lead him to the bedroom and offer him sex the way he likes it most. Your man will love feeling cared for, and you will get a rush from being so proactive and seductive.

Turn the tables

Nothing is sexier than a woman who is in charge of her sexuality. Maybe you have always played the submissive role but now want to have sex your way. You don't have to break out the latex body suit and a whip. Flirt with him, pamper him, and tease him. Then climb on top of him, flaunt your body, and tell him he is going to get laid—lucky guy.

Trust in lingerie

Make sexiness part of your daily routine— wear seductive lingerie that enhances your shape, even on a normal office day. It will be a little secret that no one else knows except you and your partner—if he's lucky. You'll find that you feel different about yourself when you are wearing sexy underwear instead of granny panties. It might even give you the confidence you need to rush home from work, undress for your partner, and drag him straight to bed.

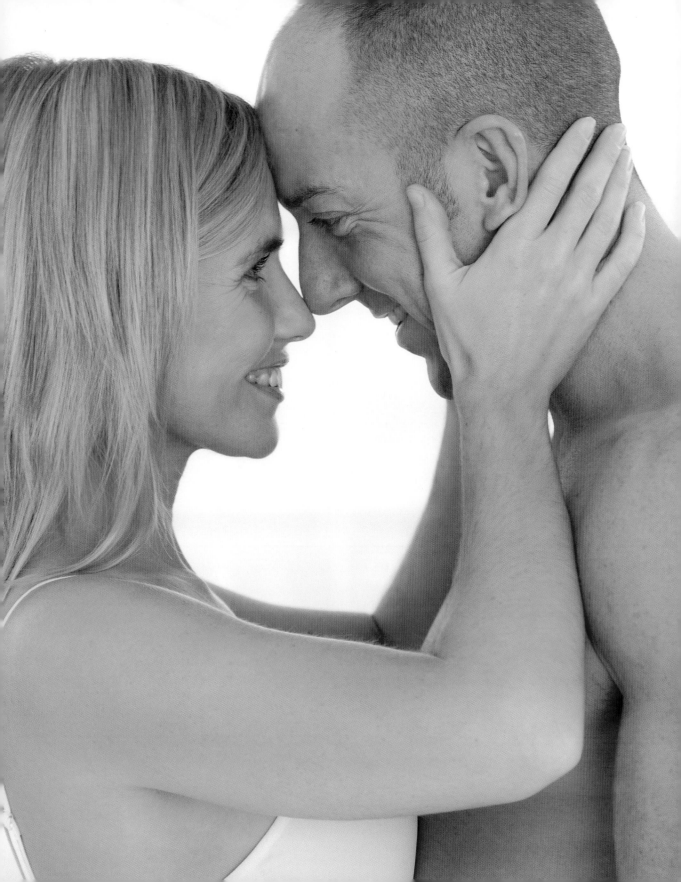

Know your relationship

Our human bonds are vital in keeping us happy. A strong, healthy relationship with a person you love and respect brings support, joy, friendship, fun, passion, and love. Yet our relationships are constantly evolving—highs, lows, and everything in between are part of our romantic journey. As both of you grow and change, you might find your relationship changes, too. At times your sex life may hit a stalemate as your career takes off or your parental responsibilities increase. The challenge is to keep your relationship fresh and sexy throughout life's many stages.

Types of relationships

Where are you in your relationship? Are you delighting in the butterflies-in-the-stomach phase, when every moment is exciting? Are you at the stage where you sleep in his T-shirt and boxers without worrying about your appearance? Or are you at the point where his minor bad habits grate on your nerves, and you long for the time when your relationship was fun, flirtatious, and sexy? Whatever the case, each stage and each type of relationship presents women with unique challenges and blessings.

Review your relationship

Romantic relationships can be incredibly varied, so a one-stop shop for advice won't work for everyone—each situation is unique and requires a different set of responses to effect positive change. In order to maintain a strong emotional and sexual relationship throughout the natural progression of your life, you need to understand where you are in your relationship and where you want your relationship to be in the future.

New relationships

The beginning of a relationship is an intense and memorable time. From your first kiss to the magical moment when you realize that you are in love, new relationships can make even the most composed person's head spin. Your libido is in overdrive, your senses are supersensitive, and being apart is unbearable. The simplest things— a whispered endearment or shared confidence— have the power to take your breath away, and every moment spent together is precious. However, as the saying goes, the course of true love never did run smooth, and many of the issues confronted by couples at the beginning of their relationship—from lifestyle habits and beliefs to interfamily relations—will set the tone for your future relationship. Communication is especially important during this phase.

Long-term relationships

Marriage and lifelong partnerships are the quintessential monogamous relationships. Most people aspire to obtain lifelong love, though divorce rates show that the journey to "happily ever after" is harder than it might seem.

Long-term relationships promise love and companionship, which most people crave in their lives. Most couples also have shared goals, such as having children, and financial commitments. The couple relies on each other in good times and bad, and feels completely comfortable together. Although this stage brings with it familiarity and security, it can also mean the end of passion and excitement, along with emerging worries and doubts. At this stage, couples still have to work hard to preserve the romance in their relationship.

Keep your sex life vibrant by trying new positions or techniques, and taking the time to flirt with, seduce, and romance each other. Fantasy, erotica, and sex toys may help to keep it exciting.

If work and other commitments mean you can't spend much time alone or have sex very often, keep your connection close with erotic touches, deep kisses, and loving hugs.

Open relationships

Some people believe that monogamy is unsuited to today's modern world. In an open relationship, both partners are permitted to sleep with other people. This type of relationship is generally built on the idea that lust cannot be governed and sexuality should be enjoyed and explored. However, it is only fair to be honest about your expectations. If you don't see a committed relationship in your future, tell your lover. If you one day would like to make the relationship exclusive, be upfront about those hopes, too.

Open relationships provide the comfort and companionship of a long-term relationship with the excitement of new love. The "butterflies" stage often lasts longer in an open relationship, as it does in a long-distance relationship. This is because the freedom to sleep around, or the distance, sets up a barrier that prevents a couple from moving on to a more settled relationship. Although many people dabble in open relationships, settling down remains important to most men and women. In the meantime, make sure you both practice safe sex with other partners and promote safer sex by being tested regularly. Always use protection for both intercourse and oral sex.

Also be aware that open relationships can be particularly difficult and unsatisfying for women. When women achieve an orgasm, the brain releases oxytocin, otherwise known as the chemical of attachment. Men have higher levels of testosterone in their brains, which may help to counteract this chemical. So protect yourself from becoming too comfortable with a partner who might not share your feelings: set limitations, and guard your emotions and your health.

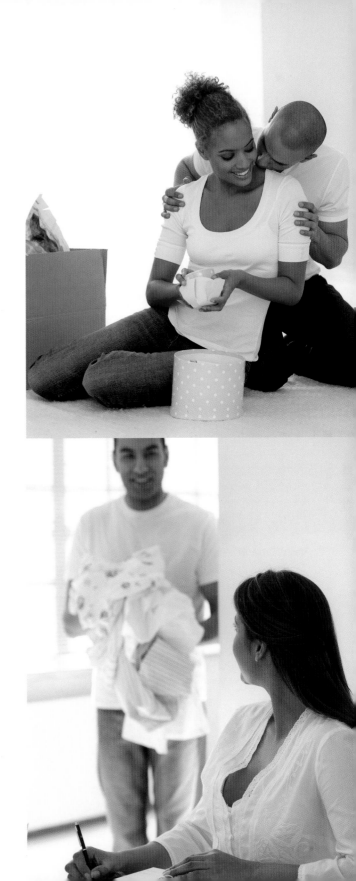

Casual encounters

These types of attachments can be temporarily fulfilling. They are often based upon sexual gratification—think one-night stands. Where do casual encounters stand in an average woman's life? Most will have explored the one-night stand at least once, and it can be tempting on a lonely night. With the right precautions, casual encounters can be a satisfying part of a woman's sexual journey.

Take advantage of the temporary situation by being as wild and kinky as you desire. After all, it's just for one night, so you don't need to hold back or feel embarrassed. Try out a new position and get in touch with your femme fatale. Casual encounters might not be the place to find love, but they can help you hone your sexual prowess.

May–December relationships

A significant age difference between partners has the tendency to set some people's heads spinning, including family members and close friends. It can also be tricky for the couple in question. With this sort of relationship, you must be prepared to confront differing age issues.

Perhaps one of you has children who have hit their rocky adolescent years, or maybe he is nearing retirement while you are just getting into the swing of your career. Different stages of life also present different energy levels and health concerns. While it is true that May–December couples learn a lot from each other, they also encounter unique concerns about aging. Age might not be an immediate issue, but will you still feel the same way when you are 60 and he is 45, or 70 and 55? How will you handle illness and aging?

Another major issue is children—whether you have them already, or one of you wants them and the other doesn't. Manage these difficulties by remembering that the relationship is not necessarily about whether you are compatible parents or whether children are in your future—shared life goals, an enjoyment of each other's sense of humor, similar interests, affection, and open communication are the basis of good relationships. If his stance on children is a deal breaker, don't force or trick him into adopting your point of view. Make a clean break and find someone who shares your dreams for the future.

Empty-nest relationships

When children grow up and leave home, one or both parents often imagine that blissful romantic nights will follow. However, many couples find that by the time they have the house to themselves again, they feel they have nothing left in common with each other. Without the children's lives to discuss, parents may find their only topic of conversation is the weather.

The empty-nest syndrome is common and expected—after all, your life is changing for the first time in 18 years. In the wake of this, your relationship will inevitably shift and evolve.

You can get it back on track, but you might have to get to know each other again. Think about building up the common ground—shared interests such as travel or golf. Now that children are no longer at the forefront of your minds, you have time to explore other interests, whether they be fitness, cooking, or gardening. While it is important to have separate hobbies to maintain your independence, having a mutual one will help create conversation and give you shared goals.

Also have honest conversations about what you want from this next chapter of your life. Take some risks by stating that you would like more intimacy, and attempt to jump-start your sex life.

These changes can herald the beginning of a new and beautiful time in your relationship—long weekends away, quiet nights, late mornings and breakfast in bed, and sex all over the house. And this really is a situation that you can create for yourselves, by yourselves.

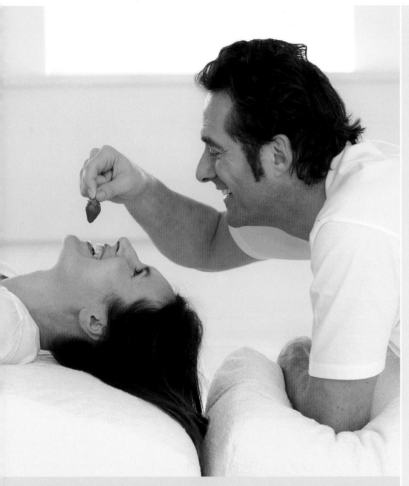

Pursue adventure

Your initial feelings of excitement when you first met your lover cannot be duplicated, but they can be imitated. When people engage in adventurous activities such as bungee jumping, riding roller-coasters, skiing, or even watching a scary movie, their brains emit dopamine and adrenaline, which are similar to the chemicals emitted during infatuation. By participating in these types of activities with your partner, you get to spend quality time together and benefit from the surges of excitement and attraction.

Stay sexy

The way we dress and groom ourselves is a large part of sexual attraction, yet many couples let their appearance fall by the wayside once they become comfortable with each other. Paying attention to your appearance reminds you, and your partner, how sexy you are. Even though you have been together a few years, making as much effort as you did on your first date can lead to similar emotional and sexual rewards.

Make a date

No matter how busy your lives and careers are, or whether you have children, all long-term couples benefit from setting a date night and spending quality time together outside the home. Go to a restaurant or a bar and spend an hour or two flirting with each other. Don't talk about work, domestic troubles, or the kids' homework. Instead, make each other laugh, enjoy kissing at the bar, holding hands in the taxi home, and having great sex afterward.

Get the romance back

Don't just long for those heady moments you experienced in the early days of your relationship—make yourselves a promise to reignite that excitement you shared together. Turn off the TV, feed each other strawberries and champagne, make love into the early hours of the morning—and don't worry if you are late for work.

Affairs

The urge to be with an attractive stranger is often a natural element of our sexuality, and striving for something new is part of being human. This is even more true when a relationship is faltering as a result of arguments, miscommunication, and unspoken needs. Affairs can create the rush of the unknown, a sense of romance, and a feeling of being sexy and desired. While infidelity is damaging, some people believe it is easier to satisfy their sexual desires with someone other than their partner.

Face the truth

As tempting as that sexy stranger or seductive co-worker may be, you first need to ask yourself a hard question: what are you looking for? Is it sex? Romance? Feeling attractive, wanted, or loved? The latter is the common response, but while you get this feeling in the short term, an affair doesn't provide for your long-term emotional needs.

Is an affair worth it? If your partner caught you or knew you were doing it, would it then be worth it? You also need to ask yourself another hard question: are you willing to do the work needed in your relationship to get what you want?

If your relationship has been under duress because of external factors, such as a change in financial circumstances, blame the issue at hand and not your partner. An affair might help you forget problems at home, but it won't solve them.

The danger of emotional cheating

Even if you remain faithful physically, emotional infidelity has the potential to short-change your partner and stifle your relationship.

Emotional cheating comes about when you devote undue amounts of time, energy, humor, sensitivity, and affection to someone other than your partner—a colleague, for instance, especially as many of us now spend more time with our co-workers than we do with our partners. We only have so much emotional energy, and if we bestow these gifts on other people, our partners will inevitably feel neglected and resentful.

Know what is real, and what isn't

You can allow yourself to feel lust for that handsome guy in Marketing. It's okay to think someone is sexy and to express those feelings in

You can even daydream from time to time that you are with a different person. But that doesn't mean you have to act on those fantasies.

private, because the more you repress your thoughts the more they will persist in your mind. You can even daydream from time to time that you are with a different person—but that doesn't mean you actually have to act on those fantasies.

Realize that what is real is the relationship you have with your partner—warts, roses, and all. If you want to get your relationship back on track, you need to put in some time and effort to make this happen. Consider counseling as you and your partner work on strengthening your relationship.

Picking up the pieces

Many people consider cheating an absolute deal breaker, but in some relationships, healing is possible. Couples' counseling is a good idea when healing. A therapist can help couples rebuild their relationship and reconnect sexually with each other, and can also help people discover why the infidelity occurred in the first place.

But to go about healing this massive wound, the injured partner will need time to vent about the way he or she feels. Couples often have a hard time bouncing back from an affair because the betrayed partner can't let go of the pain and the guilty partner feels helpless to fix the situation.

To help begin the healing process, the betrayed partner should be able to vent about his or her anger and sadness for 10 minutes a day. After the 10 minutes is up, the affair should not be discussed for the rest of the day. This will help to prevent the affair from becoming the focus of the relationship.

The cheating partner will have to be honest without being hurtful if the relationship is to make it through this period. When discussing the affair, the betrayed partner is likely to have many questions. The guilty partner should offer truthful answers, but avoid any intimate details about the other woman or man as it will only further upset their partner. Honesty is a must when rebuilding a relationship after an affair—but so is tactfulness.

Know your limits

Email, instant messaging, texts, and social networks blur the line when it comes to adultery. Sending your colleague a suggestive text or email seems harmless, but it is a form of cheating. Don't write anything in an email, blog, or text that you wouldn't say in front of your partner. At home, avoid spending hours in front of the computer when you should be with your partner. If it feels wrong, it probably is.

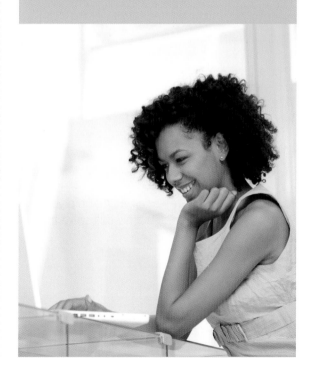

Connecting with your relationship

All relationships take work, so it makes sense that the most important relationship in your life should require the most work and commitment. "Happily ever after" is the stuff of fairy tales, but deep, lasting love is possible. It just takes effort, communication, and dedication. Luckily, the payoff is huge—a happy life, a fulfilling relationship, and unconditional love. However, it helps to know how to bypass the roadblocks, keep your love life exciting, and navigate the trials and triumphs of monogamy.

Keep it realistic

Make a commitment to reality. Your relationship isn't going to be a fairy tale. There will be times when you are not attracted to your partner, times when you want to kill him, and times when the sex isn't great. But by making a commitment to realistic goals—such as not expecting sex to be mind-blowing every time—you can create an atmosphere in which unconditional love will thrive. In addition, you will be relieving yourself of the pressure that women feel to be perfect, especially within their relationships.

Maintain the excitement

Once two people are in a committed relationship, they tend to let certain aspects of their lives fall away—sex and excitement are sometimes among them. And some couples reason that if sex isn't there naturally, you can't create it. They're wrong. By the time your relationship hits the two- to three-year mark, you need to put in some effort and use a little imagination to recreate the passion and romance of your early relationship. This might mean regular weekends away or marking a "sex night" on the calendar. But in order to spice things up, you both need to be willing.

Stay connected to each other

You love your partner, and you find him sexually attractive. But when you both get caught up in your jobs, domestic chores, routines, children, and hobbies, you can often forget to give attention to your most important connection—the one you have with your lover.

Don't become invisible to each other. Smile and be glad to see each other. Ask relevant questions about each other's day. Think before you, or he, starts ranting about work, grumbling about the babysitter, or worrying about the bills. If it is not that important, leave it unsaid. Don't waste your time on negative trivialities.

You can maintain your emotional connection by keeping your exchanges light and flirtatious. This will make it easier to feed your sexual connection—it is hard to turn on your sexual excitement when you spend the evening arguing about domestic trivia.

Eat dinner together and try to go to bed at the same time as your partner. Even if you don't have sex, you can spoon or cuddle before you sleep. Alternatively, if you both enjoy morning sex, set the alarm 20 minutes earlier and indulge in a quickie before you get up.

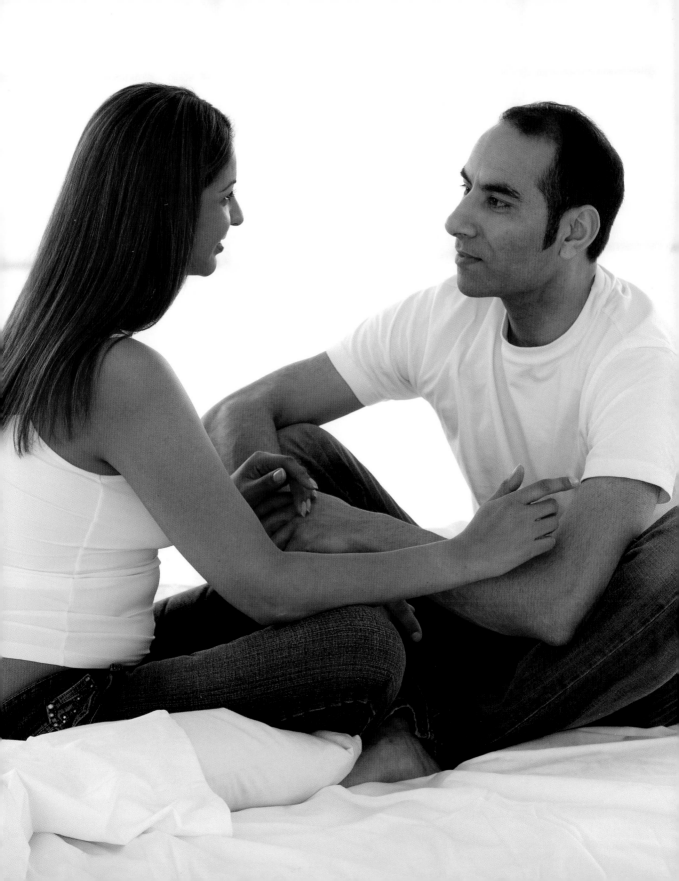

Intimacy and romance

Everybody has a desire for intimacy. Add some romance, conventional or otherwise, and your relationship becomes exciting and exclusive. We want the whole package from our loving relationships—affection, hand-holding, cuddles, sharing, lovemaking, and flowers. Though the image of a couple strolling off into the sunset is a cliché, this is what we long for. And believe it or not, it is achievable—you *can* build a relationship in which intimacy and passion abound, years after the first date.

Romance is an attitude
You don't have to wait for your lover to turn up with a bunch of flowers in order to enjoy an intimate moment. Romance is not a single event, but an ongoing attitude. When sitting in the car, reach over and touch his thigh. Leave him a love note on the fridge door. Post a sexy promise on his pillow. Call him at work and tell him you're thinking of him. These small things add up to something much bigger.

Preserve a little mystery
It might go against popular opinion, but there is no reason to share everything with your lover. He doesn't need to know that you plan to shave your legs tonight, or every sordid detail of your year abroad. He may be your soul mate and you may have the burning desire to reveal all your secrets, but a little mystery will keep things interesting. Men are usually not so inclined to share—don't demand every single last detail of his life, but do let him surprise you with the occasional new story.

Create your own moments
If your man prefers a Saturday night in front of the TV to a candlelit dinner for two at a restaurant, there is no reason why the occasion can't be romantic. Don't spend hours cooking, just order in or enjoy a gourmet takeout. Dim the lights, snuggle up on the sofa, and enjoy the intimacy. Don't let the dishes, the phone, the children, the laundry, or mundane thoughts about work interrupt your time together. Make sure you don't let the TV stop you from showing him some thigh and kissing his neck, and seize the opportunity to seduce him during the commercial break.

You are never going to agree on everything. Differences of opinion don't have to get ugly— they can even help you create extra passion.

Use your sense of humor

Make your relationship a haven for laughter, silliness, and fun. Whether it is the private nickname you call him, his shower songs, or your special jokes during sex, intimacy is created through these little secrets. Allow room for humor, even during arguments. Have a safe word you can rely on when a disagreement becomes heated—perhaps a reference to your favorite movie or a past joke he made—and agree to use it to defuse the situation. Jokes can't solve arguments, but every once in a while they can prevent a silly argument from getting any bigger.

Make disagreements work for you

Accept that even if you and your partner have almost everything in common, you are never going to agree on every single topic. Luckily, these differences of opinion don't have to get ugly—and sometimes they can even help you create extra passion. Use the heat generated from your political debates to spice up your relationship. A little verbal sparring can be very sexy, especially if you are secretly fantasizing about tearing the other person's clothes off. Your different beliefs can create excitement in the bedroom.

Your relationship can continue to be fun, intimate, and romantic—with the proper nurturing, it should be the most fulfilling and meaningful part of your life.

Reap the benefits of intimacy

The most beautiful part of being in a relationship is knowing that you are not alone—that no matter what else happens in the world, you have someone to count on to make you laugh, wipe away your tears, and pick you up when you are down. You and your partner can take turns at being the support system—when you have health or family concerns, you know you have someone to worry with you and to offer practical help. Take turns caring for each other, whatever happens.

Loving rituals

Sexual and emotional routines are a simple way to create intimacy in your relationship. Nonsexual rituals such as Tuesday-night tacos, Friday-night movies, or breakfast in bed on Sunday can help to create intimate bonds between you. You should both look forward to these rituals, and enjoy them. You can also create sexual rituals—you may already have a few, such as cuddling after orgasm.

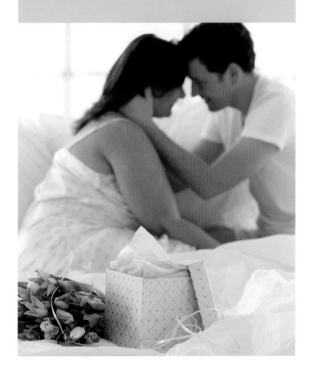

Sex files: Rebuilding sex and intimacy

Being intimate with your lover is more than just having sex; it is the way you communicate physically. This couple's problems stemmed from lack of intimacy. Their story shows how important it is to continue to treat each other as desirable, even when you don't have time for regular lovemaking.

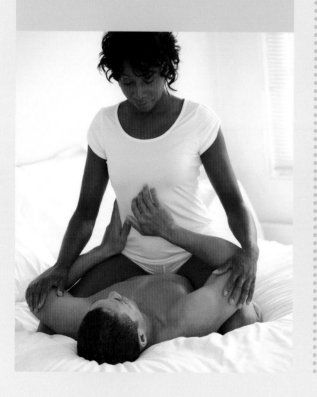

Background

Morgan, 45, and Derek, 47, have been married for 10 years. They have three children: six-year-old twin girls, Lacey and Brooke, and an eight-year-old son, Max.

The problem

Morgan and Derek came to see me after Derek had a near brush with infidelity. Morgan had discovered some private emails that Derek had been sending to a colleague. Although not overtly sexual in nature, the emails contained enough affection and emotional intimacy to make Morgan concerned. In the emails, Derek had also written about problems in his marriage, which made Morgan feel betrayed and alarmed, since he'd never mentioned any problems to her. In addition, they hadn't had sex in months, and cuddling, kissing, and affection had all but disappeared.

In my personal session with Morgan, I asked her if there had been any clues beyond a nonexistent sex life that might suggest Derek wasn't happy. "I don't know," she replied, "I've got three kids at home. The girls have been ill, and before that Max was having problems at school. I have a part-time job too." It became clear that Morgan and Derek didn't spend any time together without the kids. "We're supposed to do a date night once a week, but it never happens. Something always comes up."

When I spoke to Morgan about the emails to his colleague he explained that he liked feeling attractive and wanted. "At home Morgan ignores me and talks to the kids, or she talks to me about the kids. Or she gives me chores and then nags me about them."

Finding solutions

My first homework assignment to Derek and Morgan was for them to spend at least 10 minutes a day alone talking and reconnecting in the bedroom with the door shut. No discussion about the kids or household concerns allowed!

For their next assignment, I told Derek and Morgan to set their date night in stone since there's no point in having a date night that never happens. Without time away from the routine of parenthood and household chores, relationships inevitably suffer. A date doesn't have to be elaborate or expensive—simple things such as going for a coffee or having a picnic are fine.

To rebuild intimacy I asked Derek and Morgan to take baths together, give each other massages, and to touch each other in their daily life. By making these forgotten touches part of their routine, I hoped they would rediscover the connection and flirtation that once existed between them.

Finally I asked Derek to be aware of the times when he felt intimacy slipping—and to talk to Morgan non-judgmentally about it

rather than seeking solace away from her. I asked Morgan to step back a little from the children and spend more time with Derek—although he was a loving father and provider, part of him still needed to be celebrated and appreciated as a man.

What happened?

Derek cut off contact with his colleague, and, after just one hot bath together, Morgan and Derek ended their long sex drought. As sex returned, so did the spooning, cuddling, and tenderness that they'd both missed. Now that the channels of communication have reopened, Morgan and Derek find it easy to talk frankly.

Keep communicating

All couples experience times when sex isn't great and intimacy is lacking. The next time you feel disconnected from your partner, speak to him or her rather than seeking comfort elsewhere. Just the act of talking will start to reconnect you.

Communication

Good communication skills are the foundation of all relationships, and particularly romantic ones. Misunderstandings, crossed signals, and hurt feelings abound when communication is lacking or nonexistent. This is especially true when it comes to sex. Not everyone is comfortable verbalizing his or her needs or speaking up when something is awry in the bedroom. As a result, sexual dilemmas are ignored or misinterpreted, which may lead to unnecessary arguments.

Learn the skills

Good communication within a couple allows both partners to state their case, or talk without interruption or judgment. Being a good communicator is not just about choosing the right words and winning the argument. It is about listening to the other person and responding appropriately. Effective communication allows both partners to express their needs.

Even partners who communicate well can have problems when it comes to discussing sex. Create great bedroom communication by using verbal and physical skills to help your partner understand what you need.

Accept your differences

Men and women don't always appreciate that they have different responses when it comes to stressful situations. When confronted with a dilemma, men often switch into problem-solving mode. Women, on the other hand, tend to empathize and listen rather than look for an immediate solution. This can lead to problems when couples discuss emotional issues (including sexual ones), since both people have different expectations and needs from the conversation.

Use body language

We instinctively understand and respond to our partner's body language. We are programmed to respond to smiles, kisses, and snuggles—not to mention sexual cues. The next time your partner is doing something you enjoy, let your body talk to him. Arch your back and wrap your legs tighter around him, or lean forward to give him a better penetration angle. All these movements tell your partner what you enjoy, without you having to say a word. Eventually, he will look for these little non-verbal suggestions, so when you aren't responding as intensely, he will know to change positions or vary his speed.

Offer positive encouragement

Never complain or give negative feedback during sex unless you are in physical pain—it is sure to kill the mood and may even cause an argument. Instead, try to give your feedback in a positive way—maybe in the form of a compliment. Tell him that what he is doing feels good, but might feel even better if he tries it another way. When he understands which strokes and touches you prefer, he can cater to your pleasure more effectively—and you, in turn, can satisfy his.

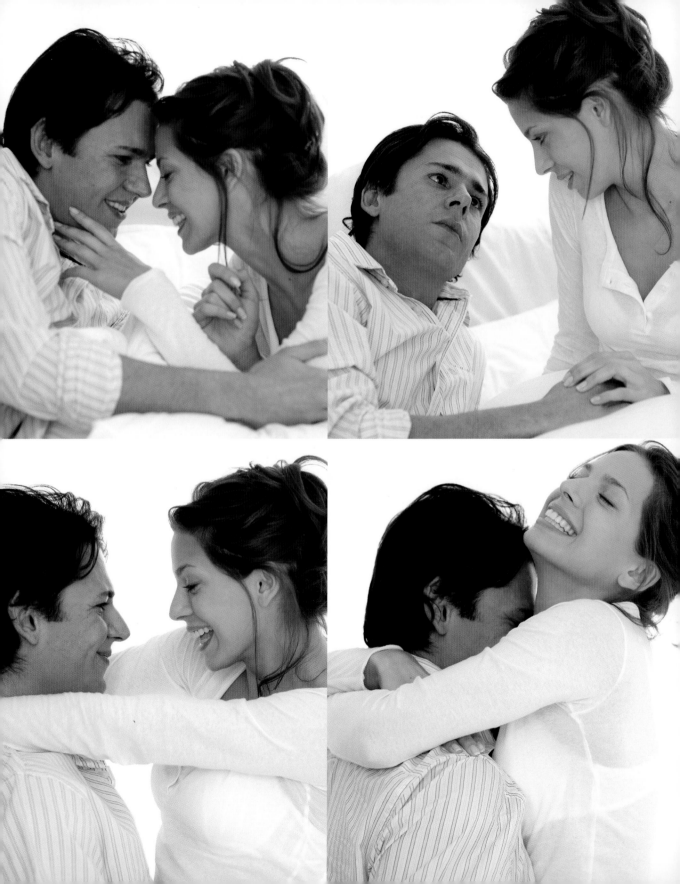

Female communication

Men and women communicate differently, which can affect their romantic and sexual relationships. It starts in childhood, when we are socialized to express our emotions and needs in distinct ways. These differences might be genetic. Baby girls tend to respond more to facial expressions and react by making cooing noises. Baby boys tend to zero in more on the mechanism of how things work. As adults, we need to work around these differences and find effective ways of communicating with each other.

Skillful communicators

Women are usually effective communicators. We are creative and skilled language users—compassionate to those in trouble and empathic with other women. We often rely on intuition when communicating with our partners.

Women are also interested in the emotional lives of their friends, colleagues, and family members. We enjoy listening and sharing. It is not uncommon for two women to exchange intimacies within 30 minutes of meeting.

In the bedroom, women can excel at warm, empathic communication and paying genuine and sexy compliments to a lover. If there's something we want to change, we have the skills to broach the subject with tact and sensitivity. We can use positive feedback and body language to communicate without criticism.

The drawbacks of empathy and emotion

Being emotionally aware and intuitive can also have drawbacks in the way we communicate. For example, we tend to protect other people's feelings, so we may not ask for something we really need or want, or we may say "yes" when we mean "no." In a sexual context, this could mean

that you don't tell your lover that you want more foreplay in case it seems critical. Or you withhold the fact that you don't like anal play.

We also tend to get emotional when we feel upset or angry, and this isn't always the most efficient or precise way to get a point across. Take the following example: you come home from work exhausted and find a pile of dirty dishes in the sink. You yell at your partner and tell him he's thoughtless. He, in turn, feels nagged and resentful. The alternative approach is to calmly explain that you take the dishes personally—as a symbol of his lack of consideration and respect. (To him, they may just be dirty dishes.) You could remind him that it's his turn to do dishes, and that you're looking forward to relaxing with him later.

Choose your moment

Women tend to be impulsive, but spontaneously broaching serious topics such as sexual or emotional issues doesn't always foster the best discussions. You have to find the right place and time to talk about them. Raising a problem when your partner has just walked in the door or is watching TV probably won't get a positive response. Bide your time and take your man for

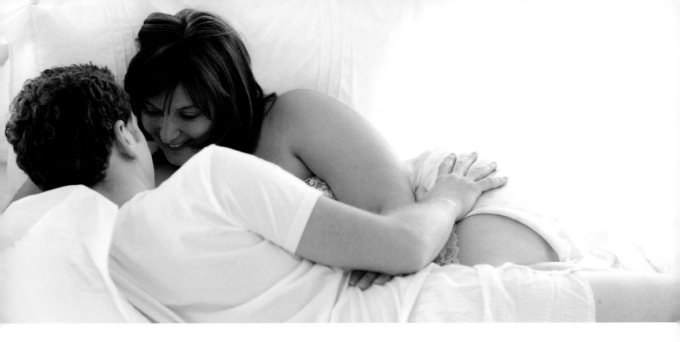

a drink or a walk in the park to discuss the subject sensitively. Similarly, if your partner wants to talk about your relationship, but the time's not right, don't put him off, but tactfully postpone it. Tell him you want to talk—and it's important to you—but you need time to relax after work, for example. Then set a time for a discussion.

Lean on your girlfriends

Everyone has their bad days, and sometimes all you want is to give in to a good, long rant. Go ahead—letting off steam allows you the release you need so you can get on with your life.

But make sure you surround yourself with the right audience. Most men aren't socialized to vent for venting's sake—they would rather offer a (maddeningly!) sensible solution to the problem at hand. And while venting might make you feel better, unbridled complaining to your partner is not always conducive to a good romantic or sexual relationship.

Think about what you are after: if you want an uninterrupted hour-long ranting session, you might find it more satisfying to call on your girlfriends—and their fabulous communication and empathic skills—instead.

Pillow talk

A common road bump when you get into a new relationship is the issue of sexual histories. Many women wonder when is the right time to ask about their partner's past, or to share their own history. This is up to you, of course, but generally it is not a good idea to talk about old partners—it is irrelevant. What is worth sharing is whether you have been exposed to any sexually transmitted diseases, and what lessons you have learned along the way. Anything else is immaterial and may lead to unnecessary conflict.

Communicating with your partner

The jokes are true—when communicating, many men rely more on monosyllabic responses, and even grunting, than actual words. But while the strong, silent type can be attractive, you might be wondering how you can tune in to what your partner is actually thinking. Why won't he tell you about his day at work? Why did he clam up after your latest argument about the bills? Look to his non-verbal cues for hints—and recognize that sometimes silence and a little space are the best policies.

Take note of his actions

If this gender gap in communication styles has you distressed, don't be. Men might not often borrow from our repertoire of feeling, but they have their own way of expressing their intimate emotions. Subtle actions like grabbing your hand as you cross the street, walking on the outside of the sidewalk, and carrying in the heavy groceries are all expressions of the way he feels about you.

For him, actions speak louder than words. He might not be much of a sonnet writer, but if he calls you when he knows he is going to be late or if he remembers your favorite takeout dish, recognize that the undertone of those actions is "I care about you and I want to take care of you."

Look for physical cues

While verbal flare-ups might be inevitable at times, you can reduce their frequency by tuning in to his unique form of communication.

When your man is in a bad mood, you don't need him to tell you. There is usually some physical representation of his distress—his jaw is clenched, his hands tightly balled up. If this is the case, don't make the situation worse. It is a bad time to start forcing him to communicate. We have all made this mistake—our partners come home in a bad mood, and all we can do is repeat, "What's wrong? Tell me. Is everything okay?" While this might be a sure-fire way to get your girlfriends to open up, it is likely to further annoy your partner and make him withdraw.

Your partner might not respond to you verbally, but he may respond to you sexually. In other words, don't take his bad mood to mean that sex is not an option. It may be just what he needs to open up to you.

Learn his language

In an argument, most men prefer to deliver their side of the conversation as shortly and effectively as possible. They don't want to discuss their feelings—they prefer to find workable answers to the problem and move on.

This type of communication can't always apply, but sometimes it is a good idea to take a lesson from his "less is more" style of talking. The longer and more drawn out that a discussion becomes, the more room there is for hurt feelings and miscommunication to occur. Keep it short and sweet—save your marathon-like energy for other more positive and fun activities.

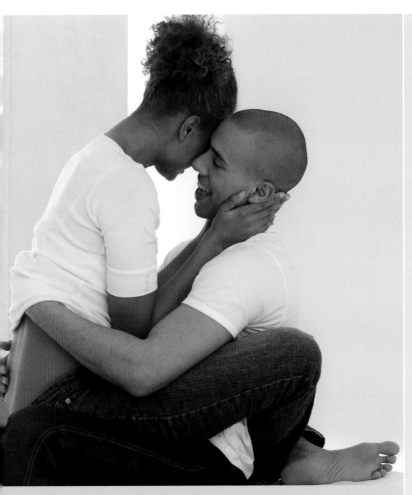

Enjoy the present

Women sometimes can't help trying to juggle a million things at once. This means that we have a difficult time staying in the present and letting go of worries about the future. Maximize communication with your partner by letting go of constant worries about what's to come, such as concerns about paying for the kids' college or impending visits from the in-laws. Instead just remain in, and enjoy, the present.

Share your worlds

Not many women get involved in their lover's hobbies, but having shared interests is one of the best ways to nurture your relationship. Even if you're uncertain about football or don't know much about the latest music, try to show an interest in activities that your man likes. In return, he can get into your world by trying golf, yoga, or Pilates. You don't have to love the same things to have a great relationship, but having mutual interests to share will keep your communication tight.

Show, don't tell

Nothing beats action when you're trying to send a message. Don't waste your breath telling him what you want sexually—lead him to the bedroom and show him the way you'd like sex to be. If you want more foreplay, murmur where he should stroke, lick, or suck your body. Similarly, if you want to try a new position, redirect the action by moving your body into position. He'll be thrilled that you are taking the lead, and happy to comply with such sexy demands.

Tune in to your man

Your partner might not be as eloquent as you at expressing his emotions, but don't dismiss him as uncommunicative. Take steps to encourage him to be more open. Sharing intimacies and goals will help. So, too, will putting minor worries in their place, and supporting his interests. And don't forget that in his world, actions are what count.

Communicating needs and desires

Most people have high expectations of relationships. We want humor, companionship, fidelity, comfort, romance, security, and shared life goals. Many of these expectations are unspoken, since people presume their partners are aware of their needs. But if these expectations are not being met, it might be time to communicate your needs and desires. Most couples encounter some communication problems, and there are some simple techniques to enable you to navigate these situations successfully.

Communication is a two-way street

Effective communication begins with a willingness to listen to each other's needs, even if it isn't always what you want to hear. You also have to agree to treat your partner in a kind, fair manner. By making compromises to keep each other happy and by offering honest feedback on your needs and desires, you both have your expectations of your sex life and the relationship fulfilled.

Communication sometimes breaks down between couples when one partner broaches a complaint and the other feels criticized or undervalued. However, if both partners agree to view each other's feedback—even if it isn't always positive—as a tool for enhancing the relationship, rather than a personal attack, communication can improve from both sides.

Talking about sexual issues

When these expectations involve sexual desire and needs, communication can be trickier. Problems with your sex life can be difficult to address, especially if you are in a long-term relationship and neither of you has ever discussed issues relating to your sex life. But the more you ignore a sexual concern—such as your need for

more foreplay, your concern that sex has become routine, or your desire to try new positions—the more the concern will grow in your mind.

Instead, find a neutral time and place—not right before or during sex—to give your partner sexual feedback. Frame it as a compliment, such as "I love it when we spend time on foreplay before we have sex" or "I love having sex with you—I think we should do it more often."

Communicating through actions

Talking about sexual attraction is not always easy, and you may discover that communicating with tact may in fact involve more action and less talk.

If you find yourself less attracted to your partner than you used to be, try to identify the roots of your waning attraction—has he gained weight or let romance fall by the wayside?—and consider honestly if you are guilty of the same. Then, instead of making hurtful accusations, start a subtle change in your relationship by being proactive yourself. For example, if weight gain is the problem, inspire your partner to be more committed to his health by buying healthy foods and asking him to join you for an evening walk. If he is reluctant, gently express your concerns while still being as forthcoming as possible. Your partner should be open to your thoughts, and willing to make positive changes. And letting him know that getting healthier will boost your sex life might be all the incentive he needs.

Effecting change in your sex life

Positive change always begins with proactive efforts. Too often, women take a back seat when it comes to their relationships and their sexual pleasure, assuming that their partners will know what they need and that the sparks will fly on their own. Unfortunately, this is hardly ever the case.

In order to create a positive change in the bedroom and in your relationship, you need to step up and take the reins. Now is not the time to be self-conscious or self-doubting—only you know what you want, and what you need. If you want more romance, don't be shy about initiating a little sexual magic to seduce your partner to your way of thinking. Light some candles, set the mood, and encourage your man to follow your lead. Along with the willingness to put in the time and effort, you also need to be honest with your partner. Let him know your needs. After all, he isn't a mind reader.

Emotionally intelligent communication

Whether you are discussing sensitive issues—such as wanting more or less sex—or arguing over the domestic chores, if you want to maintain effective communication with your partner, you need to talk like adults. This means no insults, no sarcasm, and no imitations are allowed. Instead, state your case and reasoning clearly and concisely, then actively listen to your partner's reply. Demonstrating healthy methods of communication shows respect for your partner, yourself, and each other's opinions—it is the trademark of emotionally intelligent communicators, who maintain a peaceful relationship even during disagreements.

Shared time

If you and your partner want to get your communication—and your sex life—in sync, it helps if you share some lifestyle habits to give you time to be intimate. Try to eat together at least once or twice a week. Go to bed together, and get up together in the morning. Work together on a goal or task, whether it is washing the car or giving each other a massage. Quality time together will improve your intimacy and communication.

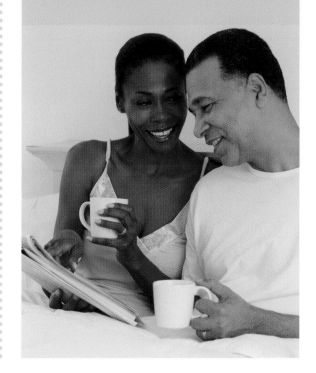

Listening and asking

Ninety percent of communication is listening. The best communicators are generally the people who take time to listen—this isn't always easy if you're on the attack, or feeling tired or vulnerable to criticism. The trick is to give your partner your wholehearted attention with the sole intention of understanding him. It's also important to know how to make requests of your partner. The best requests are made in simple, direct language and delivered without fear of rejection. But playful requests can work, too.

Learning to listen

Be aware of different types of listening, and try to catch yourself when you are utilizing a form of listening that may extend the argument and contribute to hurt feelings. Stick to involved, active listening that keeps the argument heading to a peaceful resolution.

"I'm right!" listening

Many people communicate using an "I'm right" style of listening. This is like it sounds—the whole time your partner is talking, all you can think about is how you are going to rebut everything he says because you are "right." When you listen this way, much of his communication gets lost and you never hear the point that is being made.

"Whatever" listening

When you are not engaged in a conversation because you are too tired or simply uninterested in the topic, you are not taking in what your partner is saying. This type of listening is passive-aggressive because, by refusing to give the conversation the attention it deserves, you are telling your partner that you do not care about him or his needs in that moment.

"That reminds me . . ." listening

This is when you can't listen to your partner because you are too busy going off on a tangent. For instance, he says he doesn't like your leaving the garage door open and you respond by reminding him about that time he left the dog outside all day. Your partner can't get his point across and his feelings heard because you are too busy being defensive and having a circular argument that leads back to something he did wrong. If you use digressions as a way to remind your partner of his past mistakes then the issue at hand will never have a real chance to be solved.

"I'm involved" listening

The "I'm involved" or "active" type of listening is the most effective type. When you give 100 percent of your attention to your partner, you give off a vibe that shows you are interested and involved. You maintain eye contact, nod when you understand his point, and raise questions (but do not interrupt) when you don't understand what he means. In return, he is involved in your feedback. This is the quickest and most effective way to resolve any argument, but it will take both of you to use this method of listening.

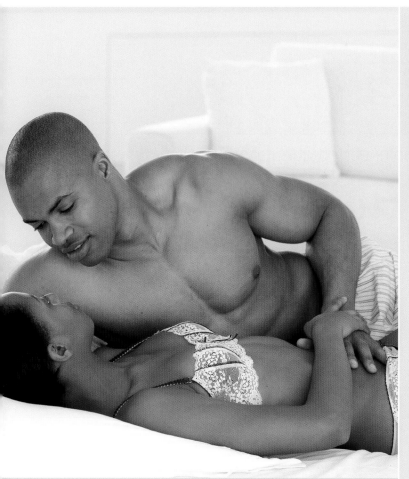

Make a game of it

Turn your sexual requests into games. Do this by literally playing a game, such as chess or tic-tac-toe. Whoever loses has to fulfill the other person's sexual requests for the night—which could be anything from play-wrestling to woman-on-top sex. Have fun. Playing games will prevent requests from becoming intimidating and will spark some seriously sexy competition.

Take turns

Spend some time swapping sexual requests. Whoever is feeling braver should go first. After he confides, for example, that he would secretly love you to talk dirty to him during sex, you can tell him, for instance, that you have always wanted to be more dominant in the bedroom. Be as specific as you can—if you want to tie his hands and feet together, tell him. Play this turn-taking game throughout the night, or take turns over a period of a week, devoting alternate nights to indulging each of your wishes.

Be accommodating

If your partner asks for something that makes you uncomfortable, don't feel forced to fulfill it. But find a way to accommodate him so he isn't discouraged from making requests in the future. For instance, if he asks you to video a sex session but you aren't comfortable with being on the small screen, tell him you would rather pretend there was someone else in the room taping. Set up your room as a faux movie set and surprise him. By taking his request seriously, you will create an atmosphere of openness and honesty.

Asking for what you want

Women often find it easier to listen effectively than to state their needs in the bedroom. It can help to make a game out of sexual requests, or to take turns with your partner in revealing your sexual wish list. And if he asks for something that you don't feel you can deliver, be creative and try to accommodate him in a different way.

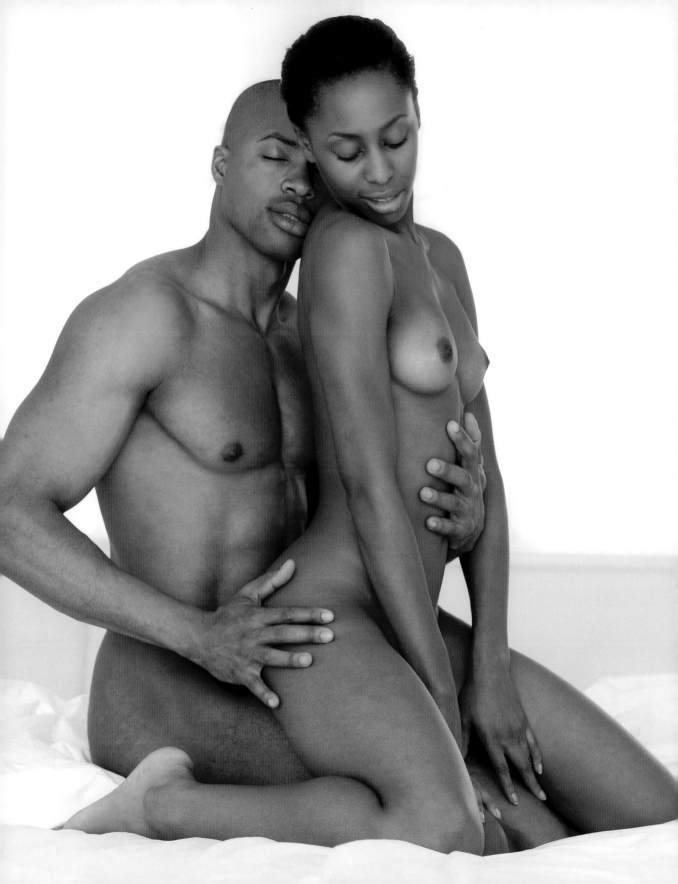

sexploration

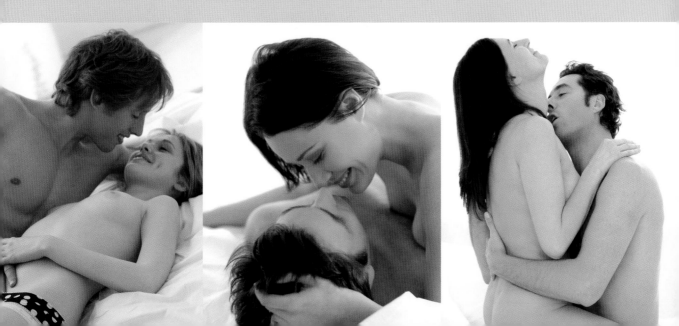

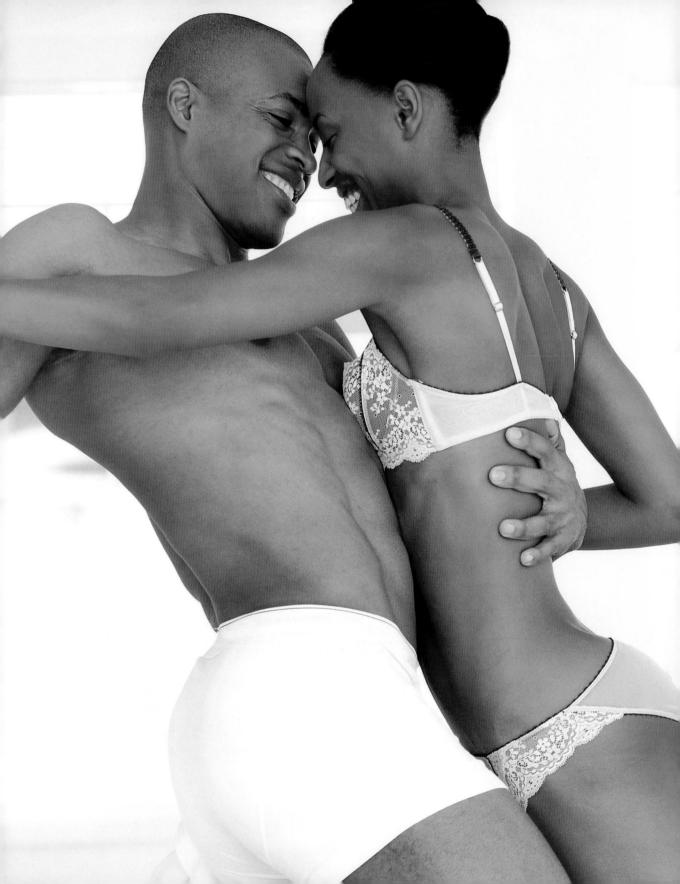

Arousal and orgasm

When did you last feel the thrill of having all your senses fully aroused? Sex is not just about achieving an orgasm—the peak sexual experience—it's about the incredibly intimate sexual journey you and your partner take to reach the ultimate pleasure. You can use your tongue, fingers, hair, breasts, or even a sex toy to give and receive an all-over-body sensory experience. So if you want to keep your sex life red hot, it might be time for you to embrace some tingling, truly orgasmic foreplay. Try kissing, touching, licking, and sucking to excite all your senses.

Kissing

If it's been a while since you shared a passionate embrace, go find your fella and kiss him deeply. You might be pleasantly surprised where it leads. Kissing is such an everyday action that we tend to take it for granted and perhaps only use it as part of foreplay. Don't underestimate the erotic power of the kiss. Smooching with your lover away from the bedroom shows you both that the sexual attraction between you is alive and kicking, and it can help to keep the zing in your relationship.

Kissing cues

From the first passionate kiss you shared with your partner to the quick peck you planted on his cheek on your way out of the house today, lip-biting, tongue-wrestling, saliva-sizzling kissing is an important part of the sexual experience for men and women. Yet while some may view kissing as merely a prelude to sex, it is actually an important bonding mechanism. In fact, many women gauge a future partner's sensual capabilities through kissing—if he's a good kisser, she predicts that he'll be a good lover, too.

What couples love

Men love kissing, and women do, too—it's a fact. For men, the more open-mouthed and deep, the better. The chemical cues in the saliva, swapped during kissing, may alert the male brain to a woman's reproductive status. But, science aside, kissing encourages deeper intimacy between you, so don't relegate it to the bedroom. For women, kissing of all kinds is good: light, deep, soft, and passionate. Next time you get the chance, let your man know how much kissing turns you on. Smooch with him to enhance intimacy, to arouse him, and to show him how hot you find him.

When your man kisses you, he is telling you that he is feeling sexy, he wants to get up close and intimate, and that only you can satisfy his passion. Accept the compliment by allowing his caresses to arouse you and get you in the mood for some life-enhancing sex.

Your very own style

However, don't be too concerned if your kissing connection isn't always sizzling. You can get your kisses back on track by giving your lover positive reinforcement and demonstrating the styles you prefer. For instance, if his kissing style is too aggressive for your liking, say "I love it when you kiss me softly and slowly"—then show him just what you mean. Or when you see a stirring kiss at the movies or on TV, lean over and whisper, "That really turns me on—let's try kissing like that."

If you are in a new relationship, asking him what he enjoys isn't very romantic, but you could find out by letting him take the lead. Are his kisses quick and intense or slow and moist? Discovering his style lets you deliver the lip action he craves—and then you can show him what drives you wild. Being clear about your likes and dislikes early on avoids problems later.

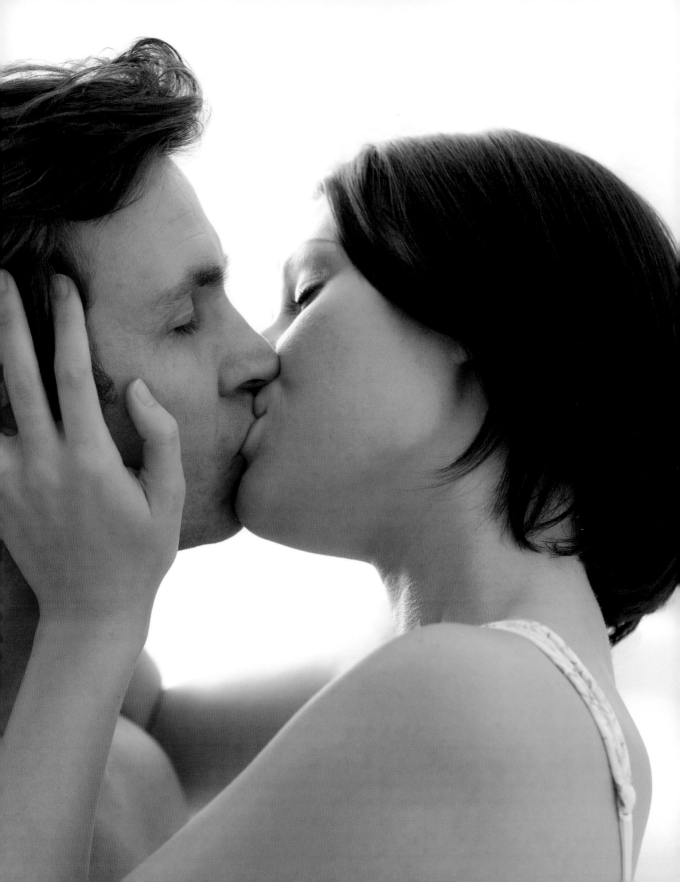

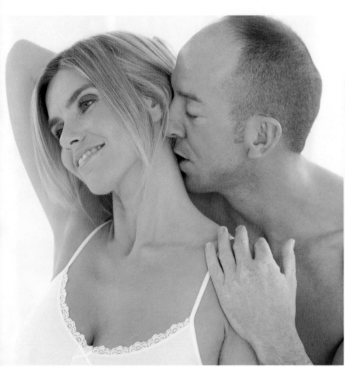

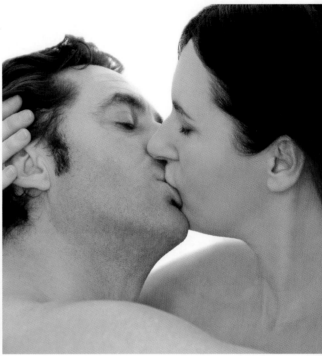

"Kiss-switching"

You can also try out a "kiss-switching" policy. Take turns kissing each other the way you most enjoy being kissed. Try sweet, soft kisses interspersed with deeper, wetter, tongue-fondling ones. Spend time experimenting. You'll both learn about the kisses the other desires and get pretty aroused in the process.

Getting back into the groove

Kissing quality is important, but so is quantity. In long-term relationships, couples sometimes find that kissing falls by the wayside, particularly during busy, stressful times, and this contributes to a lack of intimacy and spontaneity, which negatively affects their sex lives. Start by giving your partner a 10-second-long kiss every single day. It will feel weird to count to 10 in your head as you kiss, but it's merely a tool to get you back

into the habit of kissing each other intimately again. It's important to make sure you kiss each other at the end of the day or before bed, and when you say hello and goodbye to each other, but you can also surprise him with a kiss when he least expects it—perhaps when he first wakes up in the morning. Try resetting this important sensual trigger in your relationship—you'll be surprised at how romantic and sexual kissing can be when you make the effort to recommit to it.

Kissing in foreplay

Once kiss-play becomes a daily part of your life together, make sure it also plays a big part in foreplay. Kissing can sometimes take a back seat, but nothing can be sexier or more intimate than an intense make-out session. Instead of rushing through the kisses, spend a little time curled up with your lover, reconnecting to the lost art of

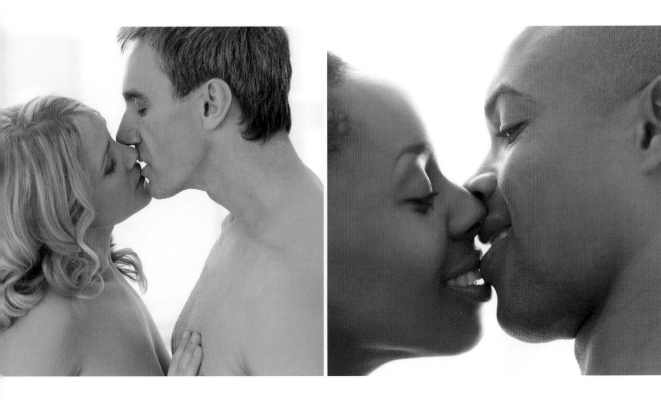

necking. Don't have an agenda to make sex the focus. Instead, just revel in the simple pleasure of kissing. Make your kissing technique direct and lingering. Don't rush, but gradually move from exploratory, light kissing, to deeper, open-mouthed movements. Explore your man's lips and mouth with your own, using light force and intention—let him know you really mean it.

Kissing during sex

When you are having sex, don't push kissing to the side. It can be an integral and sensual part of making love. Although not all positions are lip-to-lip friendly, most lovemaking is intensified with delicious making out. So the next time you are on top, try out a few different things. For example, experiment with leaning full length on your partner and slowing the pace as you share a deep kiss. You can also give slow smooches to prevent

your man from reaching orgasm too quickly. This can be effective in the missionary position. You can try initiating warm sensual kissing to slow down penetration and delay his orgasm. The best part is that kissing during intercourse heightens your connection and your pleasure, making you both more likely to reach climax.

Kissing all over

Kissing during sex doesn't have to be limited to lips. Encourage him to kiss you all over your body, while you tantalize his erogenous zones with your lips. Simultaneous kissing is especially seductive. Beware of his nipples, as they can be very sensitive, so use a delicate touch and concentrate on his entire chest area. Most men find that light ear nibbling and neck nuzzling are also very erotic, especially if you stimulate or cup his genitals as you kiss him.

Touch

Having your skin touched and caressed, and stroking your partner in return, relaxes you, arouses your senses, and satisfies a primal urge to connect intimately with another person. As the largest organ in the body, with millions of tiny nerve endings, the skin responds to pleasure, pain, vibration, heat, cold, and pressure. It is thinnest on the genitals and thickest on the palms of your hands and the soles of your feet; nerve endings are most abundant in the lips and the tips of the fingers.

A few facts about touch

Touch is vitally important for your everyday relationship as well as your erotic one because it is the cornerstone of human bonding and affection. It is one of our first sensations in the uterus and crucial for healthy childhood development. Our need for touch is fundamental to our sanity and well-being: take these signs of affection away and we suffer stress. Yet, surprisingly, affectionate touches often all but disappear in long-term relationships. All the long hugs, cuddles, and tender caresses that are constant in the beginning of a relationship are forgotten. This is generally because our need for touch is not recognized or prioritized and gets replaced by child care, work, household chores, and the million other things of everyday life. As we get older, lack of touch can be detrimental to loving relationships as well—without regular caresses and embraces, a couple's intimacy and closeness can suffer.

Source of contention

On top of this, touch may be lost in a relationship if the couple assumes that all touching has an erotic focus and is relegated to foreplay. As a result, nonerotic touches such as cuddling, light kissing, and embracing are given up. In relationships where desire is uneven (such as those where the man wants sex more often than the woman), touch may become a source of contention. The man doesn't want to touch the woman for fear that she may reject him, while she may be afraid to touch the man because she is afraid that he will think she is trying to initiate sex.

Nonerotic touch

If touch has become overlaid with confusing or negative messages, couples should establish a time for nonerotic cuddling, and then set the boundaries clearly. Regular touch will naturally increase intimacy, which may balance out your sexual needs; he will be more satisfied and you may want sex more often. Making nonerotic touch an everyday part of your relationship—playing with your partner's hair, for example, or tickling their back—can get your relationship back on track, and help create an environment in which erotic touch can be reborn.

This is especially true if you touch without sexual pressure or expectation—as with kissing, touching outside of the bounds of foreplay can be a powerful libido enhancer. Even if you're not

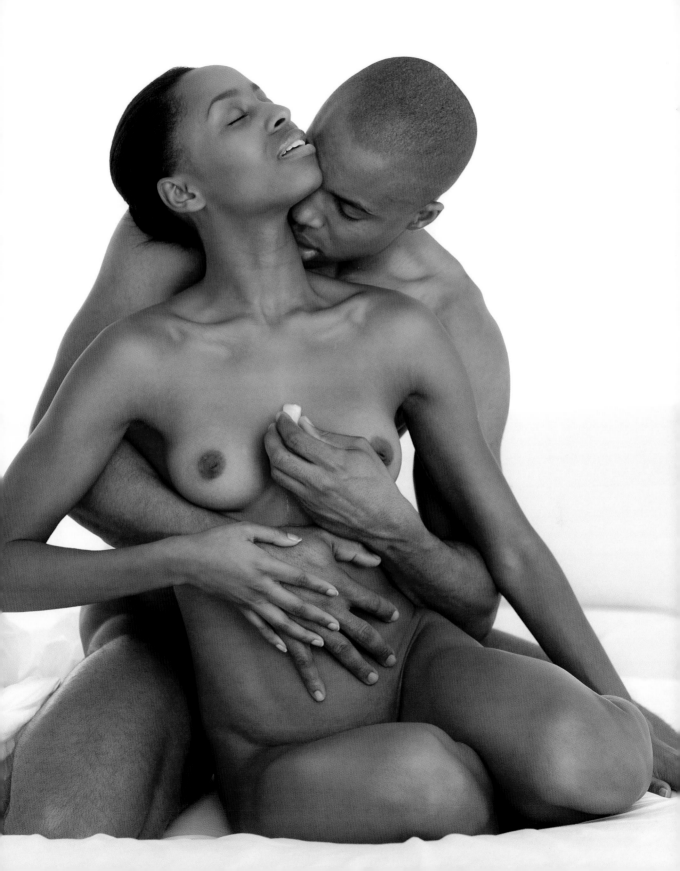

experiencing mismatched libidos, don't lose the sense of touch in your relationship. Find simple, sexy, and satisfying ways to connect physically throughout the day and night, then start using touch to enhance your erotic relationship, too.

Hellos and goodbyes

Start with a good-morning cuddle. If your schedules are different or neither of you are morning people, implement touch in a slightly different way. Greet your man from the shower with a fluffy towel straight from the dryer. He'll associate the warmth and softness of the towel with your soft embrace.

Before you leave for work in the morning, don't just throw a peck on your partner's cheek as you run to the car. Take one minute out of your busy schedule to set an affectionate, loving tone for the rest of the day. Wrap your arms around him and plant a kiss on his lips. It will have you thinking of each other all day long.

Wrestle for it

Remember back in school, when flirting meant playfully punching the boy you liked? Or when the kid who had a crush on you would pull your hair and run away? These silly, flirtatious moves often end as you move into adulthood, but a few competitive caresses can bring a little fun and sassiness back into your relationship. The next time your man crawls into bed and tries to steal all the covers, don't just whine about it—roll over and attack him with a little erotic wrestling. Rolling and play-fighting under the covers can be highly sexual, especially if you are nude.

Even if you are fully clothed, wrestling can be a powerful libido enhancer. The next time you're arguing over who controls the television remote, challenge him to an arm-wrestling match to settle the issue. Any activity that increases your heart rate and gets you into physical contact will be good for your sex life.

Sweet nights

Make your bed and bedroom a sexy, relaxing part of your home. This is crucial for setting a romantic mood and will make your bedroom a place where you and your man want to spend time. Make sure the mattress is supportive and comfortable, and has good bounce. Higher beds are better for helping you achieve different positions than low-slung beds, but you can always improvise. Choose silky high-thread-count sheets in luxurious fabrics so that when you and your partner head to bed, you will both be enveloped in soft touches.

Once you've set the bedroom scene and bedded down, think about touching him in a more primal way. For example, you could start things off by curling your fingers loosely in his hair or trailing your nails gently along his back.

Light it up

Before you actually get down to touching each other, think about just looking first. The sight of naked flesh is incredibly erotic to both men and women, and simply baring all can really make you feel like getting tactile. If you feel self-conscious, think dim lighting—candles and firelight will give your skin a warm glow. Bathe in the soft light and set about arousing each other's senses.

Try out different things

Touch is a vital part of human affection and bonding, and it can have healing powers when used often and well. Spend time thinking about opportunities for sensation in your relationship—this will lead you to be more touchy-feely. Find new ways to use gestures that convey warmth and love each day. Experiment with sensations of hot, cold, smooth, and rough. Try rubbing a piece of ice across your partner's bare torso, or heat things up by placing warmed stones on his back. These sensual experiments will naturally lead you to rethink and reinvent the sexual touches you use in your relationship.

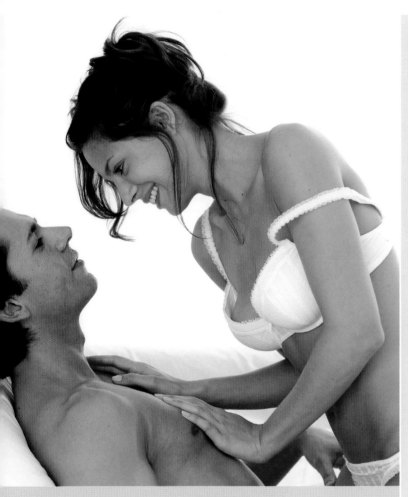

Relearning erotic touch

Invite your lover to worship your body with different types of touch. Try out the three tantalizing techniques explained here and see where they take you. Experiment with new sensations to evoke all the senses, try hug love for sweet intimacy, and use touchy-feely foreplay to get you both in the mood for some deliciously hot sex.

New sensations

Make his world melt away when you kiss him, by evoking all his senses. Look deeply into his eyes, wrap your arms around his neck, and press your body against his. Lick your lips. Kiss his lower then his upper lip. Open your mouth and run your tongue around the inside of his lips. Give him a little tongue and use your mouth to invite him to kiss you back. Now it's his turn.

Hug love

Show him how excited you're feeling by giving him a sexy hug. Press your body up against his and run your hand all the way down to the base of his spine. Caress and squeeze his bottom. Use your other hand to stroke his face and neck. Squeeze his ear lobe. Put your mouth on his, then push your pelvis against him tightly. Reach down and rub his genitals through his clothes to tell him what you want.

Touchy-feely foreplay

Use a blindfold and then set out to tantalize his senses. Trickle a little honey over his lips and then lick it off. Heat up your mouth with warm water or tea, then use your hot lips and tongue to caress and lick his hot spots. Take a silk scarf and rub it over his face and his hands, and massage his penis and testicles. Rub your naked breasts and genitals over his face, chest, and penis. Finally, drape your hair—or use a feather wand or boa—over his body and use it to tickle and caress his throat and face. Take off the blindfold, then use your new sensory knowledge to heat things up during sex.

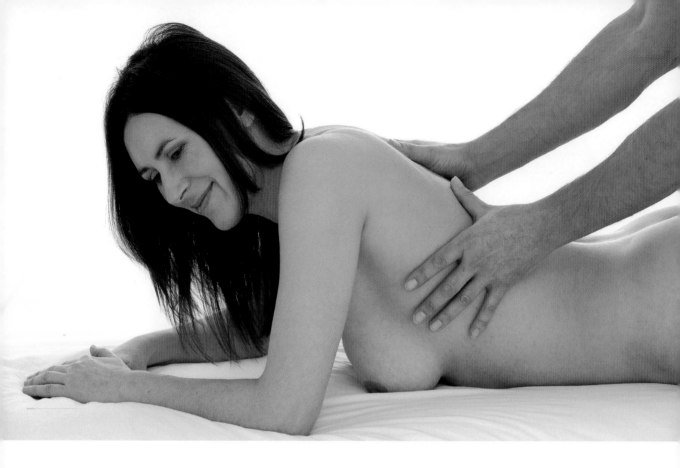

Sensual massage

Sensual massage is intended to help couples connect intimately with each other, stimulate the senses, and set the mind free. Sometimes stress or distractions coming from outside prevent people from enjoying even the best massage, so choose a time and a place in which you feel the most relaxed. Wait until you have switched off from work and the kids are asleep, then turn off the phone and spend some time getting comfortable before beginning. After this massage, you might find that you are both so relaxed and stress-free that sex naturally follows, but that doesn't need to be the end result. Relax, take it slowly, follow the basic massage techniques, and see where the mood leads you.

Starting off

◀ Before you begin, sprinkle a few drops of massage oil onto your partner's palms. Ask him to warm the oil by rubbing his palms together. He can begin the massage by running his hands over the length and breadth of your body—neck, back, buttocks, and legs. This is good for releasing tension from all over your body.

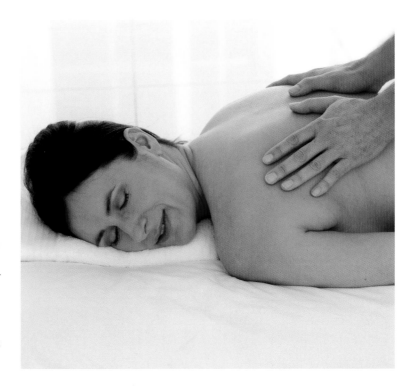

Circling

▶ A good technique to start with is circling. This is a basic massage stroke in which both hands move in circles in the same direction. The thumb and forefinger move in wide or tight circles, applying gentle pressure as they move. Your partner can imagine writing in sand and experiment with different kinds of strokes to discover which you enjoy the most.

Kneading

▶ Another feel-good technique is kneading. This is great for stretching the skin and releasing handfuls of tension from your—and your partner's—shoulders, back, hips, thighs, and other fleshy areas. Using his thumb and fingers, he can grasp an area of your flesh and alternately squeeze and release. Ask him to start at your shoulders, then move down your back to your bottom and hips. Using gentle movements, he can then knead the backs of your legs and your calves. Give him plenty of positive feedback so that he knows how much pressure to use and how much you are enjoying his touch. When it's his turn, remember that he will like to feel a bit more pressure than you.

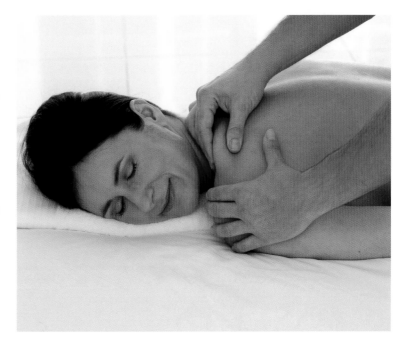

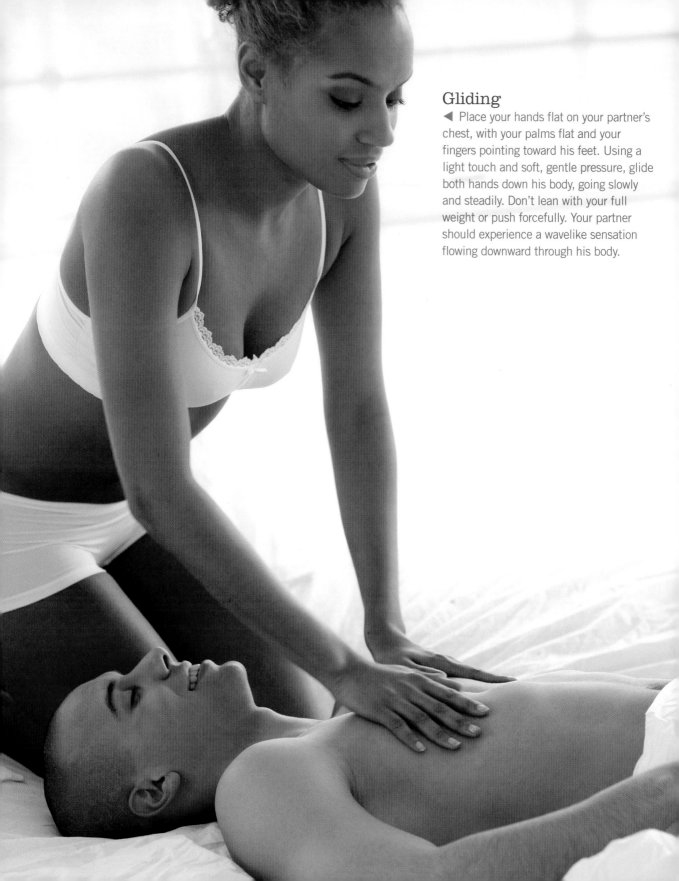

Gliding

◄ Place your hands flat on your partner's chest, with your palms flat and your fingers pointing toward his feet. Using a light touch and soft, gentle pressure, glide both hands down his body, going slowly and steadily. Don't lean with your full weight or push forcefully. Your partner should experience a wavelike sensation flowing downward through his body.

Thumbing

▶ Thumbing is a technique to stimulate pressure points on the back that promote overall well-being. Have your man gently cup your torso with his palms, while resting his thumbs on your spine. He can then run his hands up the length of your back, applying gentle pressure with his thumbs. In this position, he can also "walk" his thumbs down your spine, gently massaging each vertebra as he goes. Ask him to use a light touch because your spine can be quite sensitive to massage.

After this massage, you might find you are both so relaxed that sex naturally follows. Take it slowly and see where the mood leads you.

Feathering

▶ The final stages of a good massage should include feathering. Ask your partner to softly drape his fingers across your back to create a light, almost imperceptible touch that will send shivers down your spine. Now switch places so that he has a chance to experience the delights you've just experienced at his hands.

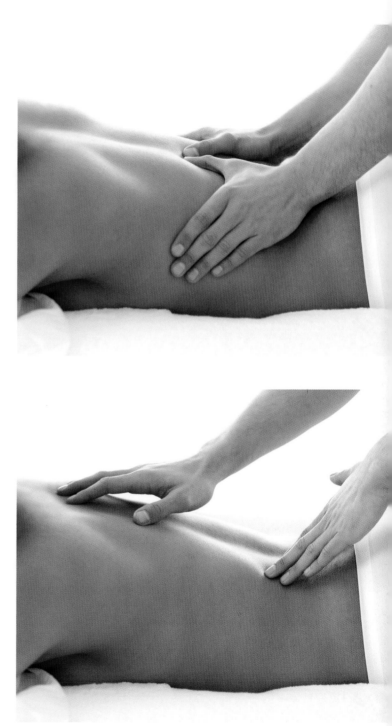

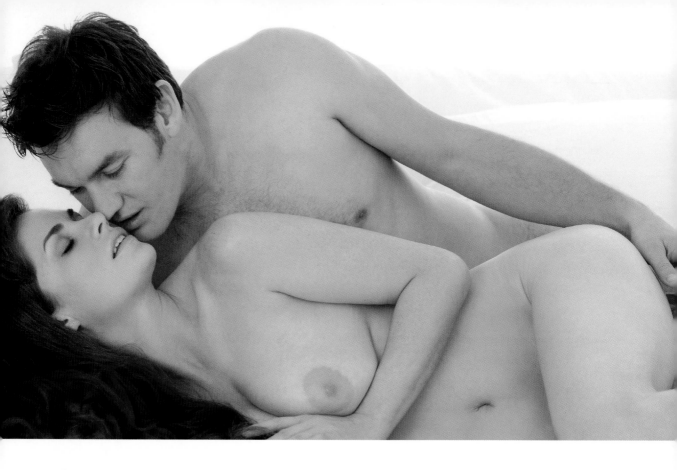

Erotic massage

This is sensual touch at its most exciting. Unlike traditional massage, which relaxes and unwinds, erotic massage stimulates the receiver's nerve endings and the giver's senses, and will leave you both feeling hot and sexy. This type of massage is an excellent form of foreplay. Kiss, touch, and massage to create an all-over-body sensory experience. Surprise each other with new types of touch. Focus on obvious hot spots like the genitals, breasts, and bottom, but also target the inner thighs, lower abdomen, and other sensitive places. Finish by playing with the idea of happy endings—erotic massage, just like any form of prolonged foreplay, can lead to more intense orgasms.

From behind

◀ Get into a spoons position, so that you can kiss and nuzzle. Ask him to smooth his hands down your back and side. When he gets to your bottom, suggest he reach between your legs and gently massage your labia. When you're feeling aroused and wet, he can massage your perineum. If this is a new sexual experience for either of you, let him gently massage your anal region with one well-lubricated finger—lie back and enjoy.

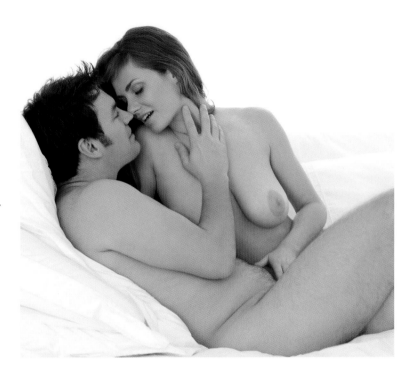

Down under

▶ Kiss and nestle while massaging his genitals. Run your fingers down his chest and gently cup his penis and testicles before massaging them. Don't make an orgasm your goal. Instead, keep your touch light across his genitals. Keep him aroused by applying constant, but nondemanding, pressure so he doesn't reach orgasm too quickly.

Chest play

▶ Ask your man to trail his fingertips delicately over your body. Ask him to cup your breasts with his hands while he kisses your neck and nuzzles your ears. When he moves on to massaging your breasts and nipples, ask him to keep his touch light and gentle, as nipples (both men's and women's) have lots of very sensitive nerve endings. He can use his other hand to rub your labia and clitoris. Not only will you be getting turned on, he will also get to admire you as he arouses you with his hands. Just make sure you keep telling him what feels good and encouraging him by giving him plenty of positive feedback on his technique.

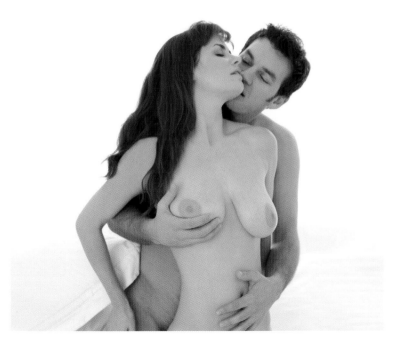

Understanding arousal

Orgasmic sex starts with arousal. Many experiences are equally arousing for men and women, but there are some gender differences in the laws of arousal. Women are often aroused through mental stimuli, such as flirtatious conversation or seductive reading material. Men, on the other hand, prefer visual or physical stimuli, such as the sight or touch of bare skin. Different sensory experiences create different responses, so it's all about finding what turns you—and your partner—on.

The signs of arousal

When we are aroused, our bodies change in both perceptible and imperceptible ways to prepare for sex. As we respond to kisses and caresses, we go into the "excitement" phase— breathing becomes shorter and faster, and heart rate increases. Some women also find that their breasts swell slightly and their nipples become erect. If you continue being aroused, you move into the "plateau" phase. Your vagina swells and becomes lubricated, while your man's penis engorges with blood. Your cervix even rises slightly, in preparation for lovemaking.

The "climax" phase is when intense feelings of pleasure begin. Your genitals contract and you experience a sense of euphoria. Finally, you move to the "resolution" phase—breathing and heart rate return to normal and blood flows away from the genitals, which return to their pre-sex state.

Mindful arousal

Unless you are in a very new relationship—when you are in an almost constant state of arousal— most people find they need a little time to turn on their sex drive. This is particularly true after a stressful day at work or at home. Both sexes need to be shown they are attractive, so a little flirting, kissing, and cuddling should be on the menu. This time allows both of you to relax and get in the mood, so keep it slow and pay attention to your lover's body language.

Purposeful pampering can also play a big part in foreplay for women. A long bath, a session at the beauty salon, and even a workout can boost a woman's confidence and her libido. Women find it hard to become instantly aroused and may worry about distractions, whereas men tend to be less discriminating—they don't care if the dog is barking or your legs are unshaven, for example.

Easy gratification

However, even if you're not in the mood, you'll probably find that your body responds to your partner's advances. If he's turned on at the sight and feel of your tousled, unwashed early-morning self, why fight it? Next time you wake up to your man's caresses, don't run for the shower. Revel in the spontaneity of sex without foreplay, and find room for a quickie. Candles and rose petals are nice—but they are not always realistic, so accept the less romantic but still sexy "must have you now" version that your partner loves so dearly.

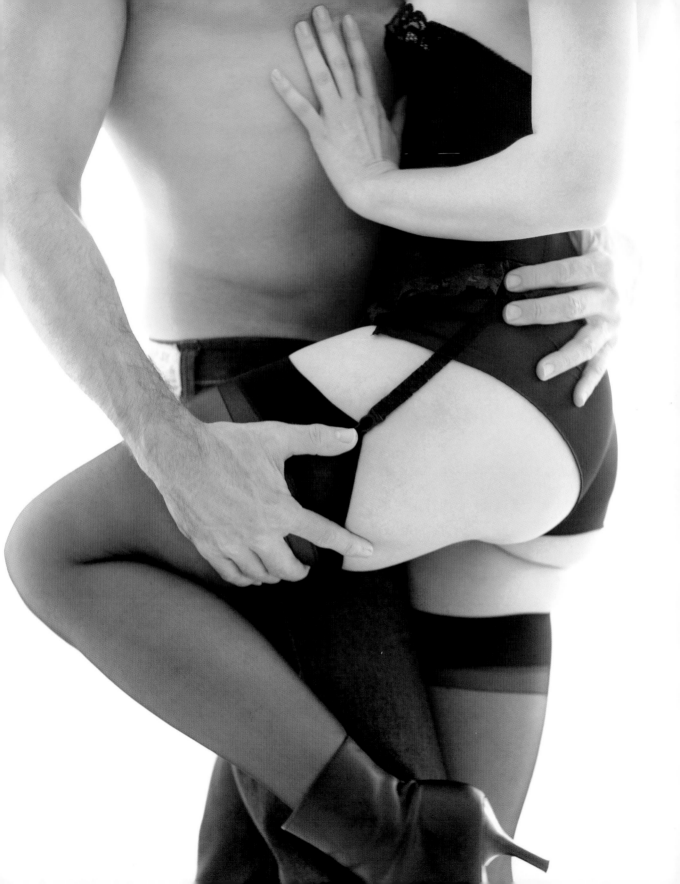

Female arousal

Women are complex creatures, so it's not surprising that sometimes we find it hard to just flip a switch and get in the mood for sex "right now." This doesn't mean we are not aroused by the same stimuli as men. Watching a sexy movie, thinking about a favorite sexual fantasy, or watching a semi-naked guy walk down the beach turn us on. Arousal is instinctive for men and women, but women sometimes need an extra step—a sincere compliment or a sensual kiss—to get turned on.

Everyday arousal

An underlying factor in female arousal is that sex begins way before the bedroom. In other words, if nothing sounds sexier to you than a long bath, a nice dinner, and freshly laundered sheets, you are probably a woman. It might not be easy for him to understand, but sometimes the sexiest thing your partner can do is to help you cut down on your to-do list, so that you can have the space, time, and energy to really focus on sex.

Peak arousal

While some men can become aroused and get an erection in just a few minutes, women can take up to 30 minutes to reach their arousal peak. So take your time and make sure that foreplay is on target. Men often don't realize that women need extra stimulation to reach a state of arousal where they can achieve an orgasm.

You might want to be treated to a little luxurious body stroking, some gentle massage, and perhaps oral or genital play to get you ready. This is particularly true if you have been faking orgasm (a big no-no). If so, you will need to start afresh and tell your partner what moves you need to really get you in the mood.

Ask to be aroused

If you want extra foreplay, try treating your partner as you wish to be treated. Slow things down by performing oral or manual sex on your man, and then ask him to do the same.

Set the scene with candles and music, and make foreplay the focus of the evening. If your partner still isn't addressing your needs, don't be afraid to spell it out for him. Men like directness; they are usually not very good at picking up subtle clues, such as the fact that you've changed your hairstyle, bought new underwear, or had your nails done. To increase the time you spend on foreplay, start by telling him what turns you on.

If you are seeking a change in the bedroom—such as the addition or removal of a certain technique or position—use positive reinforcement instead of complaints. Tell your partner, "I love it when you stroke me softly and slowly—it makes my whole body come alive," or "I love it when I get to take control and be on top. I love to see the pleasure on your face." Any type of positive reinforcement is sure to stick in your partner's head and help him to focus more directly on what gets you feeling aroused—and he won't even realize that the whole thing was your idea.

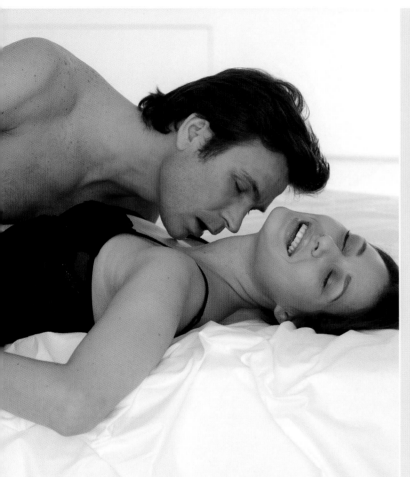

Head massage

It feels wonderfully sensual when your scalp is massaged at the hair salon. Your partner can recreate this pleasure by gently playing with your hair or caressing your scalp, stimulating a series of nerves whose effects you will feel all over your body. Ask your lover to kiss and stroke the nape of your neck as well—the area is rich in nerve endings and stimulating it can be deeply arousing.

Nipples and breasts

How you like to have your torso, breasts, and nipples touched is individual to you. Encourage your lover to experiment with different types of touch. He can use his mouth, lips, tongue, or even his penis to gently rub and caress you into arousal. Some women love having their nipples sucked, and even gently teased with their partner's teeth and tongue. If you enjoy this, tell him so. If not, ask him to use his hands and fingertips to lightly massage your breasts and nipples, using light swishing touches and strokes.

Scratching and biting

Using your nails and teeth is considered to be deeply erotic in the *Kama Sutra* and it's worth spending time experimenting with different types of mouth- and finger-play. Ask your partner to lightly scratch your upper arms, your back, and then your inner thighs. Encourage him to gently bite your neck, your chest, the backs of your knees, and your palms. Nerve endings are the key to pleasure, so get him to go for those sensitive spots that crave touch.

Pleasure places

The best compliment you can pay your lover is to show him how his touch arouses you. Encourage him to focus on new erogenous zones: head massage can be sweetly sensual; having your nipples and breasts touched is an obvious path to arousal; or a nibble on the neck might be more to your taste. Try a mix of touches to see what gets you in the mood.

Female orgasm

Our intricate sexual response affords us an added bonus: women are multiorgasmic beings. Unlike men, we do not require a refractory period so don't need to rest between orgasms. As long as we continue to be stimulated, we can have multiple orgasms. The trick is to remain aroused. Once you slip back into a non-aroused state, it will be harder to get back to that orgasmic place. The clitoris is hypersensitive after orgasm, so indirect clitoral stimulation can make you most likely to climax again.

Types of orgasm

Women are capable of having three different types of orgasm, depending on the stimulation. Hot spots include the clitoris, G-spot, and cervix, and they are each capable of bringing their own type of pleasure to play. Now, aren't you glad you were born without a Y chromosome!

The clitoral orgasm is perhaps the most commonly known (and achieved) type of orgasm, and most women find it to be the most powerful. It is experienced through direct or indirect stimulation of the clitoris and surrounding area, including the labia majora.

In addition, some women experience an intense vaginal orgasm. This occurs (for some women) when the G-spot and cervix are stimulated. You'll need to find the right angle, and may need deep penetration, to stimulate your vaginal hot spots. This type of stimulation can be incredibly orgasmic, but you'll need to be fully aroused to enjoy the intense sensations.

A blended orgasm is the best of both worlds, and usually occurs when a woman's vagina and clitoris are stimulated at the same time. Positions that allow your partner to stroke your clitoris as he thrusts are good for achieving orgasm this way.

Positions for orgasm

Not all sexual positions lend themselves to female orgasm. For example, rear-entry positions usually mean that the penis misses the clitoris entirely. The best positions afford you both clitoral and vaginal stimulation, which allow for blended orgasms. Women-on-top positions are well-loved for this reason, because they allow you to control the angle and depth of penetration.

Don't be discouraged if, like many women, you find that sex alone doesn't cut it. Needing extra stimulation during intercourse is perfectly normal, and any position that allows you, or your partner, to rub your clitoris—or use a small vibrator— will help you achieve sexual gratification more quickly and regularly. Alternatively he can use oral sex or some creative handwork to give you an orgasm before or after penetration.

Sex-giving exercise

Your body needs regular exercise to help it maintain muscle control and strength. Frequent physical activity also helps keep your skin and nerve endings in good working order because it improves blood circulation around the body. But did you know that the same is true for your vagina? Without exercise, it can lose elasticity and strength—which means that your sexual response and orgasms can be negatively affected.

One of the easiest ways to heighten your orgasms is to tighten your pelvic muscles and strengthen your pelvic floor through Kegel exercises. You can isolate your pelvic floor muscles (also known as pubococcygeus, or PC muscles) by attempting to stop your flow of urine mid-stream. Do not try this repeatedly, as it can potentially cause a urinary tract infection. Alternatively, locate your pelvic floor muscles by inserting a finger into your vaginal opening and then trying to clench your muscles around your finger. Squeeze your muscles several times rapidly, then repeat the same exercise more slowly. Practice your Kegels at regular intervals throughout the day to strengthen your vagina. You can also try practicing your Kegel exercises during sex for especially intense orgasmic pleasure.

You can also purchase weighted and non-weighted vaginal exercisers to insert into your vagina to exercise your pelvic floor muscles. These are the perfect tools for women who want to strengthen their pelvic floor after childbirth, or for women who simply want to become pelvic floor pros in the bedroom.

Core exercises

Vaginal tone and pelvic floor strength can also be perfected through a regular workout of your transverse abdominals. These form the deepest layer of abdominal muscles, which run like a band around your entire torso.

By exercising these muscles, you will achieve more than just a flat stomach—you'll acquire better posture, a strong core, and a strengthened pelvic floor. Core exercises, Pilates, and yoga can help you make the most of these muscles. Engage in any one of these forms of fitness regularly, and watch your body increase its potential for orgasm.

Female ejaculation

Female ejaculation isn't a myth, but the phenomenon is not often discussed, so many women feel embarrassed when it happens and think they've urinated. A woman's ejaculate has a similar chemical make-up to semen (minus the sperm). It varies in taste and smell, depending on the menstrual cycle, and is generally a clear liquid. A woman can ejaculate a teaspoonful or a cupful!

Female ejaculation is generally achieved by massaging or stimulating the G-spot. To experience its powers, find a position offering the right stimulation, friction, and deep penetration. Your lover will need to build up pressure on your G-spot as he thrusts, while either of you stimulates your clitoris at the same time. As you approach and reach orgasm, push out hard with your pelvic floor muscles rather than squeezing in, as most women naturally do. The trick is not to hold back, and to practice.

Male arousal

According to urban myth, men think about sex every three minutes. The truth is they're not necessarily having thoughts about the sexual act, but they are having thoughts of a sexual quality. For instance, they may see an attractive woman walk down the street and wonder what her breasts look like without a bra, imagine how her bottom feels, or think about her being naked. But each man is different, so it's important to discover your partner's sexual cues and what type of arousal he prefers.

Fast-track arousal

When it comes to sex, men are usually sprinters, easily stimulated and ready to run the lap as fast as their legs can pump. Once finished, they need to rest before they can perform again. Women, on the other hand, are marathon runners—it takes us a while to get warmed up, but once we get going, we can last for hours and hours.

This might explain why all your man needs to become aroused is the merest glimpse of you taking off your shirt or bending over to scrub the bathtub. It doesn't matter how mundane the activity—the sight of your bare skin is the number one way to get his heart racing.

Flesh versus bones

Whatever you might think to the contrary, the perfect, fashion-thin body is not the sexiest thing to most men. Just as women are attracted to muscle-bound guys because they think they'll be able to protect them, men are often attracted to full breasts and fleshy hips, because they are signs of a fertile, healthy woman.

Ask your man what he thinks is sexy and he'll probably be glad to divulge what he wants to see. His fantasies will likely include two ingredients:

you and lots of skin. Keep an open mind as you listen. If he wants you to dress up in stockings, a garter belt, and heels, think about indulging him once in a while. Seeing his arousal levels peak at your display of skin is a wonderful way to boost your body image and to keep you both satisfied in bed.

Instant gratification

It's not uncommon for men to be unaware of the different gender preferences when it comes to arousal. If your man wants to skip romance for a quickie or cut to the chase and miss out on foreplay, make a point of granting his requests from time to time. He can teach you a thing or two about letting go and enjoying sex in its most raw and natural form.

He will also adore being seduced by you, so don't always leave it to him to initiate sex. Next time you're in the mood, don't stifle your natural urges; instead, pay him the greatest compliment by telling him that you want him right then. Guide him to the bedroom—or your location of choice—and enjoy spur-of-the-moment, uninhibited sex. Spontaneous sex is a guaranteed way to keep him—and you—at an optimal arousal level.

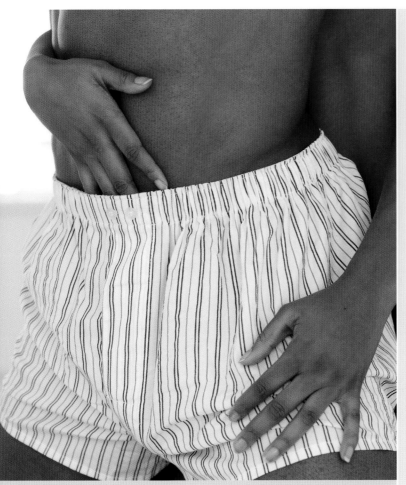

Get naked

Indulge yourself with some sexy underwear, then invite your man to a private viewing. Dim the lamps, bare a shoulder, or show him some thigh. Tell him you're feeling hot and ask him if he'd like to undress you. If you've been together a while, removing your clothes will reawaken the thrill of the first time. If you want to make it more exciting, tell him that he can only use his teeth. By the time he gets down to your sultry new undies he'll appreciate your effort and be desperate to get his hands on all that skin.

Use the whole body

Lick his chest and massage his nipples— even a little playful nipping, biting, and scratching can be fun. Draping your naked body over his will awaken all kinds of sensations for both of you. You can also excite nerve endings by stimulating him with different types of touch. Try running a feather wand delicately down his back, or use your fingernails to lightly trace a trail down his abdomen. Alternating circular and linear motions will keep him guessing about what type of stimulation comes next.

Erogenous zones

Try these fun and sexy experiments to entice, arouse, and excite your man. Put on some cheeky underwear and have him undress you bit by tantalizing bit. Stimulate his whole body with playful touches and soft caresses. Add another element by trying a new sensual location. Take charge and be creative—it won't take long to get him in the mood.

Add another element

Touch feels different when it happens somewhere other than the usual location. Taking your man to the shower or hot tub will heighten his sexual pleasure when you massage his hot spots under water. Using different vibrations from the shower head can also be arousing. If you aren't in the mood to get wet and wild, try a warming lubricant to create different sensations.

Male orgasm

Like female orgasms, male orgasms are multidimensional. When a man is aroused the sperm is drawn into an area just below the prostate, where it awaits release. This stage is followed shortly by ejaculation, and then the necessary rest-and-regroup phase. The older a man gets, the longer the rest period he needs between ejaculation and another erection, although keeping blood flow in the area (such as with a warm, wet washcloth or massage) can help a man achieve erection again sooner.

Achieving orgasm

Do men and women experience an orgasm differently? Scientific evidence suggests not: having asked a group of men and women to write down their experiences of orgasm, researchers were unable to tell, once all the gender-specific references had been removed from the responses, whether the writer was a man or a woman. So the way your man feels during orgasm is probably very close to your own orgasmic experience.

Multiorgasmic exercise

It is actually possible for a man to become multiorgasmic, too. To achieve this, he will need to master control of his pubococcygeus (PC) muscle. This will enable him to have "dry" orgasms, in which he attains the sensation of having an orgasm but without ejaculation—which means he can keep his erection and continue his arousal stage. In order to accomplish this, men can perform Kegel exercises in much the same way women do.

Finding and exercising the muscles is very similar to the process you use—he can isolate them by stopping and starting his urine mid-flow. Once he finds them, he can clench and release them throughout the day, whenever he thinks of it. Encourage him to use these muscles during sex and you can promise him that he will last longer and have more powerful orgasms.

Stop-and-start sex

Kegels are not the only way to prolong and enhance a man's orgasm. Men who struggle with maintaining their erection for an extended period of time or climaxing too quickly might find that using the "stop-and-start" technique will help to improve their sexual performance. Your man should use this technique when he is very aroused, but before he reaches climax. At this point, he should stop, pull out, and allow himself to calm down before entering you again.

If ejaculation is 10 on a scale from 1 to 10, a man should try to get to a 4 or 5 and then calm down. He should then become aroused again, almost to the point of ejaculation, but then go back down to a 4 or 5 again. By continuing this arousal and de-arousal practice, a man can gradually train himself to last for longer and experience stronger orgasms. If he finds it difficult to slow things down when he gets too close to orgasm, try to take breaks from intercourse with mini make-out sessions and other types of stimulation in order to keep him aroused and engaged, but not too close to ejaculation.

Enhancing his orgasm

Your partner's orgasmic experience can be affected if he has insecurities about his body or bedroom technique. This is one area where the emotional side of sex comes in for men—their sense of confidence is closely tied to how much pleasure you both receive between the sheets.

Enhance his enjoyment by giving him compliments on his technique and engaging in positions that are especially prone to give pleasure. Good ones to choose are doggy style and the missionary position, because they cause your vagina to clench naturally, which creates more friction and results in deeper orgasms. Try switching techniques and positions, too. A change in pressure and rhythm can delay—and subsequently intensify—his orgasm. It will also give you time to catch up to his aroused state and experience some orgasmic pleasure of your own.

Something for the weekend

You may like to try out some of the sex toys that are readily available these days and easy enough to use once you get the hang of them. Cock rings, once made of ivory, were invented in ancient times to achieve longer-lasting erections and more powerful orgasms, and today have come back into use. A cock ring traps the blood in a man's penis and makes his erection appear larger and feel harder; it will also prevent him from reaching a climax right away. This delayed gratification can make his orgasm very intense.

It is important to find a ring that fits perfectly—too big and it won't stay on, too small and using it can be painful and even dangerous. It is a good idea for a man to start by using a silicone ring rather than a metal one, and to work slowly but surely toward improved orgasms.

Does size matter?

To most women, the size of her lover's penis is completely unimportant when compared to everything else. It really is what you do with it that counts. But try telling him that.

Rest assured, size need never be a roadblock to orgasmic pleasure. It is important to your man's ego and pleasure that he feel his equipment is the perfect fit with yours. But while many couples struggle with size issues, almost all of them can be accommodated with a little creative positioning.

Believe it or not, too big a penis can be a problem. You might fear that it won't fit. Don't worry—a vagina is an incredible creation. If it can widen enough for a child to come out, it can handle an extra-large penis. Minimize discomfort with lubrication and lots of foreplay, which will increase your arousal level and maximize the potential for you both to experience orgasm.

Mutual orgasm

Some women may question whether mutual orgasm even exists—or if it is merely something that women who fake orgasms have created in their male partners' minds to massage their egos. While shared orgasms have likely been staged often, rest assured they are quite possible and can happen regularly throughout your sex life. Don't place too much importance on how and when these happen—but when they do come your way, revel in the pleasure of one of the ultimate sexual experiences.

Squeeze to please

For couples who are intrigued by the concept and want to explore mutual orgasm, it is important to begin by practicing your Kegel exercises. Control of your internal muscles will help intensify your orgasms, and clenching and releasing your pelvic floor muscles can also help you get into an erotic rhythm with each other during lovemaking.

When you feel that you are about to reach orgasm, you can help him along by tightening your muscles to let him know that you are almost there. Your man can do the same—when he feels he is about to ejaculate he should squeeze his PC muscles hard. Often, just knowing that you are about to reach orgasm will take you and your man to an orgasmic level together.

Mutually satisfying positions

The best positions for couples to achieve a mutual orgasm are probably those where one or both of you have a free hand. Maximum arousal is key, so caress your clitoris while he penetrates you with his penis. It will increase his pleasure, as he will love seeing you being so free and open. If his hands are available, ask him to reach down and rub your clitoris or your perineum.

This can also slow him down—whenever he feels like he might be near the edge, he can stop thrusting and reach down to stimulate you. Most positions allow you to do the same for him, too—reach down and tug gently on his testicles, or massage his anus or perineum, but beware: he won't be able to last long after that.

Any position in which you can introduce a sex toy will heighten the pleasure for both of you. During penetration, place a small vibrator on your clitoris. He'll enjoy the sensations it creates, too, so it may prove good for both of you.

Enjoying the sexual path

Lovemaking is the ultimate exploration and enjoyment of the senses. Experiencing mutual orgasm should be thought about in the same way. Don't make orgasm the ultimate, must-have goal during sex or you will stress yourself out and make sex less pleasurable. Besides, you will be unlikely to reach orgasm in that state of mind.

It is healthier for your love life if you can take having an orgasm out of the equation, and ask your lover to do the same. Just enjoying the journey can often lead to better sexual satisfaction and a healthier love life.

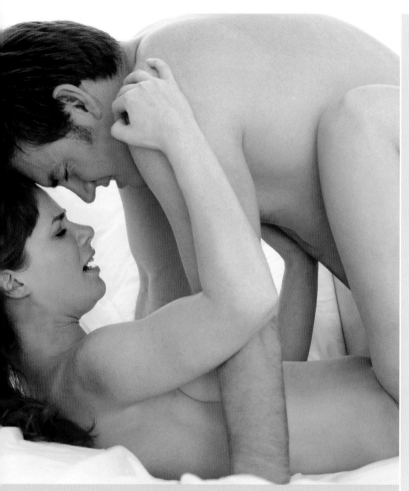

Make it different

Using a few props can take your usual lovemaking positions to the next level in pleasure. Sex toys may seem the obvious choice, but sometimes a well-placed chair or a couple of pillows are all you need to create sexual sparks. Try making love in different places, such as against a wall, on the kitchen counter, or lying or sitting on the stairs. Any place or position that changes the angle of penetration and creates new sensations will feel exciting and orgasmic.

Sex code

Encourage each other to wait for the other to climax by introducing a secret touching code. You can decide on a prearranged signal that lets one of you know when the other is close to climax. For example, if you feel you are at the point of no return, give your partner a gentle tug on his ear lobe to let him know. Alternatively, try a whispered word, a light kiss, a nuzzle on the chest, a fingernail scratched down his back, or light breathing on his neck.

Orgasmic moves

There are a lot of things you can do to make shared orgasm more likely. Try out the three ideas here to see what difference they make. A few props will help you vary lovemaking positions and take you to a different level, while having an agreed-upon sex code will let you communicate more easily. Lastly, oral stimulation may really help you both.

Oral benefits

To achieve mutual orgasm you'll probably need to experience a variety of stimulation. If you enjoy oral sex, then priming both of your responses with the "69" position before moving on to penetration can really get the sexual juices flowing. Pay lots of attention to his frenulum while he stimulates your clitoris and G-spot with his tongue. When you are both almost at the point of no return, assume your favorite position for the most fulfilling mutual satisfaction.

Sex files: Trying too hard in bed

It's possible to try too hard to impress your partner with sexual acrobatics. If you don't connect emotionally, you may misjudge what your lover wants and needs in bed. This woman felt insecure about her age and tried to compensate by having frequent high-intensity sex with her partner.

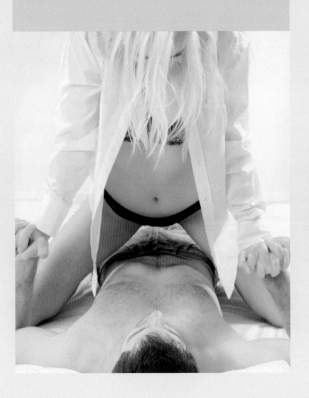

Background

Nicole is a 36-year-old executive at an ad agency and Kahlen is a 26-year-old web designer. They've been dating for a year and for the most part their relationship has been happy.

The problem

Nicole started to accuse Kahlen of flirting with other women and not spending enough time with her. Kahlen got angry because he felt that Nicole was needlessly jealous and should trust him more. They had frequent sex and were very experimental in bed, but Kahlen complained he found their sex life "over the top."

During an individual session with Nicole, I tried to get to the bottom of her mistrust of Kahlen. She said that she had no real reason to be jealous and she'd never been cheated on. She was usually a trusting and easy-going girlfriend, but once she started dating Kahlen, the 10-year age difference made her feel insecure. To compensate for these emotions, she tried to impress him sexually. "I just want to be sure he has everything he needs at home. I know I go overboard—once I tried to push him into a threesome because I thought that's what he secretly wanted."

Nicole talked about how frustrated she felt. "I'm so in charge in every other part of my life, but with Kahlen I'm out of control. I can't make him love me or stay faithful to me, so I act like a porn star to stop him from fantasizing about anyone else."

My individual session with Kahlen was also very revealing. He said, "I would never cheat on Nicole. I tell her that every day, but it's not enough. Whenever we go anywhere, she accuses me of checking out other women. Then we go home and she wants these crazy sex sessions. Even when I try to make it soft and slow, she wants to ramp it up—it feels like we're on stage."

Finding solutions

To heal the disconnection between Kahlen and Nicole, I suggested that they each make a detailed list of their fantasies (both sexual and nonsexual) and share them with one another.

I also talked to Kahlen and Nicole about the importance of connecting emotionally and sharing insecurities in a non-accusing way. If couples lose emotional intimacy, they're in danger of relying on gender stereotypes and myths to try to understand each other. In Nicole's case, she believed in the myth that "men love porn star sex and want sex all the time."

What happened?

Nicole was surprised and thrilled to discover that some of Kahlen's fantasies included very simple, sweet things, such as

"I want to go camping with Nicole and have sex under the stars" and "I want to be a father one day."

Kahlen was pleased to learn that Nicole's list was also filled with simple, romantic requests, such as "I want love notes and roses, and kisses and cuddling on the sofa".

Once Nicole realized that Kahlen wasn't secretly dying to be a swinger or a promiscuous rock star, the pressure she felt to perform was lifted. She said: "Before now I was never able to enjoy sex. I was so busy trying to be a fantastic lover I couldn't lie back and feel the sensations and the intimacy. Now Kahlen and I can have sweet, meaningful sex or wild, uninhibited sex depending on how we feel."

Talk about your desires

Never use sex to cover up insecurities or to control your partner. Talk to your partner calmly about your feelings. Ask each other about your sexual needs and desires, and really listen to the answers— that way you won't base your sex life on misunderstandings.

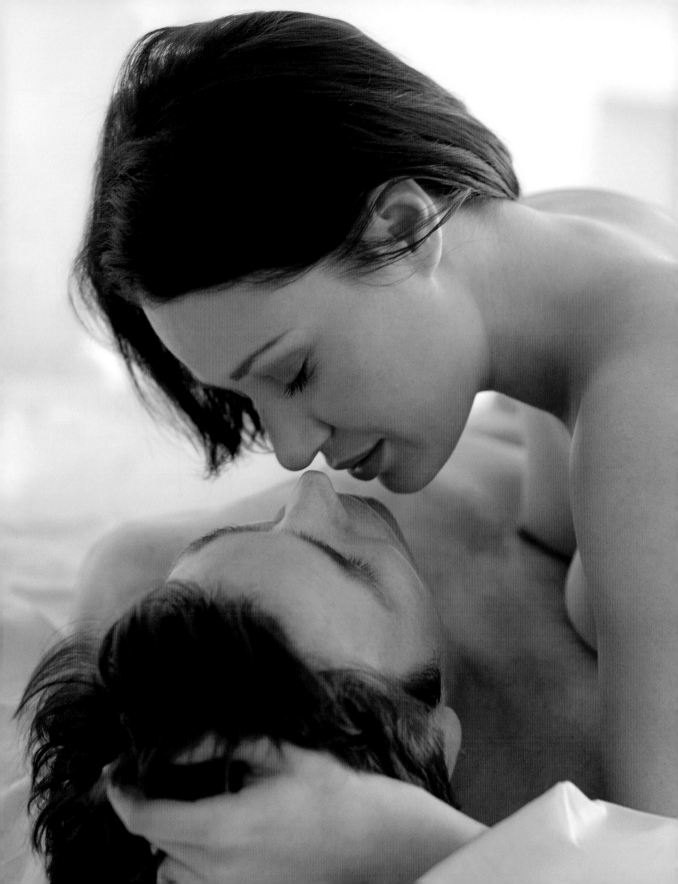

Sex essentials

It's time to bring the sexiness back into your love life. Even if your relationship is intimate, passionate, and highly sensory, you may sometimes feel like your sex life doesn't quite match up. Rebuild your sexual foundation with classic moves that you both find irresistable. Learn more about his sexual cues from oral sex, and help him discover yours with orgasmic hand-play. Then get up close with poses that put you face-to-face, back-to-front, on top, and underneath.

Manual sex

The steamiest sessions need not include penetrative sex—sometimes hand-play is the sexiest way to take your (and your man's) breath away. Few sexual acts are more intimately sensual than stroking each other's genitals. The art of manual sex can be difficult to master, because we are all different and we all have our individual likes and dislikes when it comes to genital touching. Learning how to pleasure each other will lead to enhanced confidence and enriched orgasms.

Pinpointing pleasure spots

Manual sex makes an exciting change, since it allows you to explore your sensuality and then pinpoint, before pleasuring, all the hot spots on your partner's body. It is also good to use during quickies, when you may not have the time to go to the bedroom or get undressed. It gives you both far more control as well, and you will get a better chance to discover what turns you on.

Manual techniques

Sometimes it's hard to figure out where erotic massage ends and manual sex begins, so both of you need to experiment sensitively. If this is uncharted territory, listen to each other and pay attention to the other's likes or dislikes. Let him know what moves work for you. If you would like him to pleasure your perineum and clitoris at the same time, speak up! When it is your turn, use plenty of oil and long, steady strokes.

When to use manual

Manual sex is a useful tool to have in your sexual repertoire since it can help keep intimacy alive when penetrative sex is off the menu. It can also be the stuff of erotic fantasies. Maybe you and your partner want to enact a sexual fantasy about having a teenage-style make-out session in the back of a car, or perhaps you like the idea of your partner secretly watching you masturbate in the shower, then joining in. Whatever your desires, manual sex will help tune your lover into the caresses that pleasure you most, help you understand his favorite strokes, and best of all, prolong foreplay and increase your arousal levels.

Pre-sex preparation

Everyone has their own taste in manual sex techniques, but for every couple there are some general practical guidelines that apply. Men should make sure that their nails are clipped, short, and smooth, and both of you should take all your jewelry off, as even the smoothest ring can irritate or scrape delicate skin. Most men, and some women, prefer to use a water-based lubricant, since the genitals can become dry and sensitive after repeated strokes.

Once you begin, always make eye contact when you are stroking your partner, give positive feedback, and show each other how much you enjoy being touched. This kind of communication is the best part of manual sex.

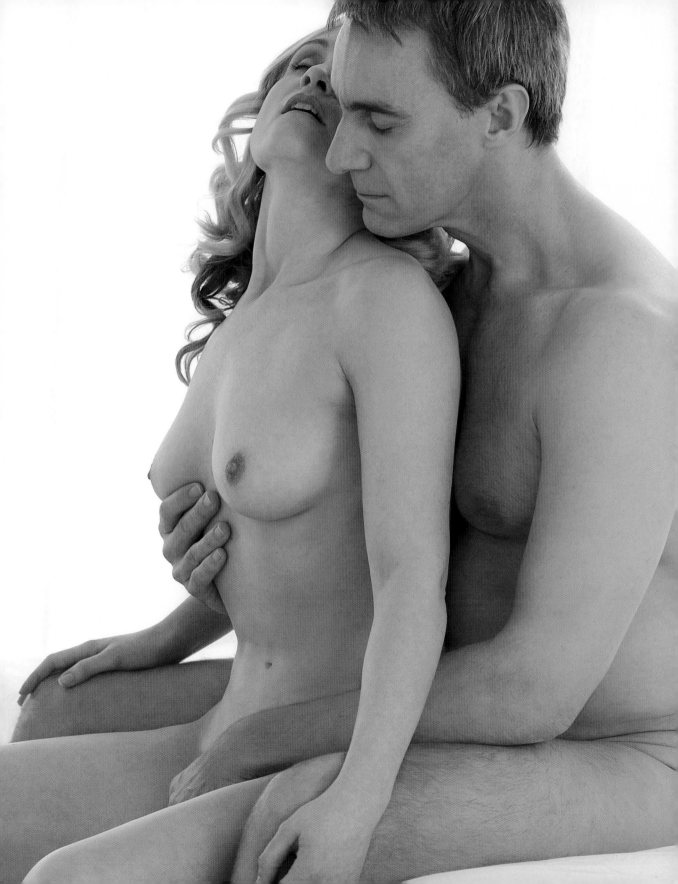

Hand-play for her

Manual sex is important for women and it can be a truly orgasmic experience. This is because it often hits hot spots a lot more easily than penetration does, making it easier to achieve orgasm. However, you'll probably need to show or tell your partner just what gives you pleasure—be sure to speak up if his strokes aren't hitting the spot. Most men just want to satisfy their woman, so by telling him what you desire you'll be letting him become the lover you both want him to be.

Your hot spots

Women have erogenous zones all over the body, and it's most pleasurable if your partner caresses lots of different areas—such as your neck, thighs, and breasts—before he starts on genital massage. When you relax and start to enjoy it (which he should be able to gauge by your secretions, body language, and breathing patterns), then he can move on to stroking your clitoris.

Clitoral stimulation

Indirect stimulation of this spot is often the most arousing, since direct touch can feel too intense, and can sometimes be almost painful. You might have to rein your man in from full-contact pressure, and encourage him to become an expert at all types of indirect stimulation.

This might include gently stimulating your clitoris with his fingers through your panties, or using his entire hand to rub across the expanse of the vulva—since your clitoris is covered by the labia you will feel sensations less directly. He can also experiment with different types of stimulation, for example by wearing lacy lingerie as he strokes your genitals. The sensations these fabrics bring might just become your new favorite sex trick.

Two-handed technique

For even more intense pleasure, you could ask him to use both hands simultaneously. This will allow him to access multiple points of pleasure all at once. The following hot spots all yield fantastic sensations when stimulated in combination: the pelvis and labia; the perineum and the vaginal opening; and the clitoris and G-spot—expect waves of orgasmic bliss.

He'll also need two hands on deck if he wants to explore your anal area while simultaneously massaging your clitoris (once his hand has touched your anal area it shouldn't go anywhere near your vagina or urethra). Simultaneous anal and clitoral stimulation can be a fast track to orgasm for some women.

Show him what you like

Use your body as a way of guiding him and telling him what you like. Try tilting or dipping your hips to encourage him to move his hands into a better position—he will quickly catch on to your body language and instinctively alter his hand movements. You can also offer to demonstrate the type of stimulation you prefer, or guide his hands with yours for some sexy show-and-tell.

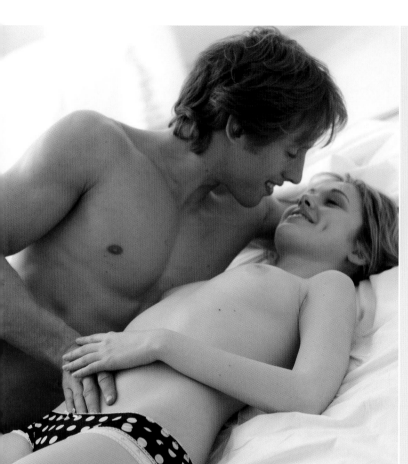

Clitoral stimulation

Take your time over these strokes. Your man needs to spend a while stroking your body before heading to your genitals. Let him stroke your inner thighs and massage your labia. Once you're feeling wet and fully aroused, then move his hand to your clitoris. His index or middle finger is more than enough to stimulate this little hot spot, and the pressure he applies is up to you. When he gets into a groove you enjoy, show him how much you like it.

Vaginal massage

Your vagina is full of highly sensitive nerve endings. He'll love the wet sensation on his fingers, so move his hand to rest between your legs and let him feel how aroused you are. While he fingers you, move his other hand to gently rub and stroke your clitoris. Together, find the speed and the motion you like best: try clockwise, counterclockwise, or back and forth, or play around with a combination of all these moves.

G-spot

To turn up your pleasure factor, give him a sexy demonstration of how to stimulate your G-spot. Make it a show by opening your thighs wide to give him a great view. Now, make a come-hither motion with your index finger, then slip it inside your vagina and make the same motion to find your G-spot. Now it's his turn. When he hits the spot, make sure you let him know. For the deepest orgasm, ask him to apply pressure to this sensitive spot and massage your clitoris at the same time.

Getting sexy

Invite your lover to discover your intimate erogenous zones using just his hands. After a warm-up kiss or two, guide his hand between your legs. Get him to make your clitoris and vagina the focus of his erotic tour, but ask him to explore your G-spot too. If he doesn't know how to find it, follow the instructions opposite for a very sexy tutorial.

Hand-play for him

It can be intimidating to perform manual sex on a man—after all, most men are already experts at self-stimulation themselves. While it's true that men are likely to be the professionals in this department, it doesn't mean that your partner wouldn't love a little helping hand. Not only does this allow him to sit back, relax, and enjoy being stimulated, it also means that he can watch you touch him, which is beyond sexy. Learning to manually pleasure him will teach you a lot about how to be his ideal lover.

Getting in gear

If you feel that your knowledge of getting your man in gear for sex is a little limited, then it might be time to brush up on the fine art of the hand job. Knowing how to find and stimulate his hot spots is a good place to start.

Make him feel like a king

Timing is important. A great moment to tantalize your partner is when he is sitting on the couch and you are beside him. Even better if you are bored and there is nothing to watch on television. For example, you could flirtatiously unzip his trousers. Make eye contact and smile a little—let him wonder what you are up to. The anticipation will make him go crazy. Alternatively, you could approach him while he's lying in bed. Just make sure that he's comfortable and relaxed before trying out your moves, and, remember, do everything with a sense of playfulness.

Heating up his hot spots

When men masturbate they tend to forgo a slow and sensual build up in favor of fast, intense penis stimulation—the time taken from first touch to ejaculation may sometimes be a matter of

seconds. So, by slowing things down and making hand-play seductive, you can offer your lover an entirely different manual experience to the one he is used to. Lingering strokes on erogenous zones such as his belly and inner thighs—both tantalizingly close to his penis—will turbo charge his arousal levels and by the time you touch his penis he'll be thoroughly warmed up.

Hand-play is enhanced by knowing about the most sensitive parts of the penis—the glans and the frenulum. By applying pressure to his frenulum (a fold of soft tissue on the underside of his glans) you can speed up his progress to orgasm. The opening at the top of the glans is also highly sensitive—he'll love it when you rub your thumb gently over the top.

Anal massage

When you're building up a repertoire of manual techniques, don't forget to include the anal area (but ask first since not all men feel comfortable with this). If your lover is new to anal touch, go slowly and gently. However, if he doesn't have any reservations, massaging his penis with one hand and his prostate with the other—using a finger inside his anus—can create a powerful orgasm.

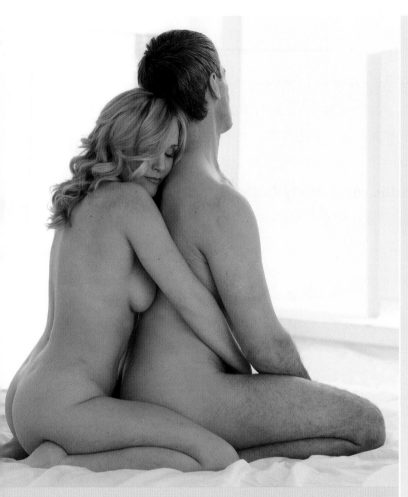

For his pleasure

If you're a manual-pleasure virgin, it helps to have a variety of strokes to offer. Try the three explained here and settle on the one that you're most comfortable with—and the one that makes him bounce off the walls. And don't get too hung up on technique: a steady rhythm, a confident grip, and plenty of lube will pretty much guarantee his pleasure.

Tried-and-true

This classic technique is loved by most men. Take one hand and place it at the base of his penis. Slowly bring your hand up the shaft, using your thumb to massage one side of it as you go. When you reach the top, immediately start massaging up the shaft with the other hand. Repeat this hand-over-hand motion until—well, you know when.

Twirling

Take your hand up, down, and around the expanse of your lover's penis. Rub slowly up and down as you would normally, but then occasionally add in the twirl—this is when you twirl your hand on top of the head (glans) of the penis. Take care not to do this too hard—imagine you are gently opening a doorknob. As you twirl, let your fingers glide across his frenulum.

All-hands-on-deck

Wrap both your hands around your man's penis as though you are holding on to a gear shift. Lock your fingers together and keep your grip comfortable, but not too loose. With one hand twisting to the right, gently twist the other to the left. Move both hands slightly up and down as you twirl and massage them around the penis. Your lover will feel as though every inch of his penis is being indulged. Continue your manual stimulation and further his pleasure by descending a little to the anal region. With your index finger, gently massage his perineum while continuing to massage his testicles with the rest of your hand.

Oral sex

Oral sex is an intimate act of trust and love between a couple. It is deeply arousing for the receiver and involves all the senses of the giver, who kisses, licks, sucks, and caresses the other to orgasmic bliss. Oral sex has always played an important role in our sexuality, and many different historical and spiritual texts tell us this. The male and female secretions are traditionally believed to have life-giving properties and the fact that orgasms are good for us means that oral is good for our total health.

The benefits of oral

Getting close to your lover's genitals brings you very close to his sexuality, which is a highly sensual, deeply arousing experience for both of you. It builds on the benefits of manual techniques in that it allows you to use very targeted pressure and movements, but gives you even more intimate contact with each other.

Men usually don't need too much persuasion to give or receive oral. Yet, despite its unrivaled potential to give pleasure, many women put this at the bottom of their list of sexual favors. If you are wary about oral, try thinking about it as an opportunity to learn more about your and your lover's sexual preferences. Be brave, turn out the lights, and enter into it with a generous spirit. You don't have to "deep throat" him, porn-star style, since the head of the penis has the most nerve endings. Start here and see where it takes you.

Techniques to try

To maximize pleasure, whether you are giving or receiving, it is essential to find a position that is comfortable for both of you. When you are receiving, open your mind to enjoying the sensations of your partner kissing, licking, and sucking your labia, clitoris, and vagina. Tell him when it feels good, and gently redirect his stimulation when it feels too intense.

When giving oral, take your time sucking his penis and licking his perineum and testicles. Switch between different speeds and pressures. If you get tired, take a break and stimulate him with your hands instead. Try taking turns. Most importantly, tune in to his moans and body language so you get to know what touch he really likes best. He might just surprise you.

Extra-sweet oral

To maximize your oral pleasure, it is worth paying a little attention to what you eat and drink. Foods such as kiwi, celery, and pineapple can make your genital secretions even sweeter. If you are worried about hygiene, try oral sex in the shower, so both of you are really fresh.

Food can work as an erotic prop in your oral games, too. Apply whipped cream and chocolate sauce to his penis, then lick off your calorific cocktail. Trickle a little honey or raspberry sauce over your genitals and invite him to savor the extra sweetness. Treats like this will make these oral sessions even more irresistable.

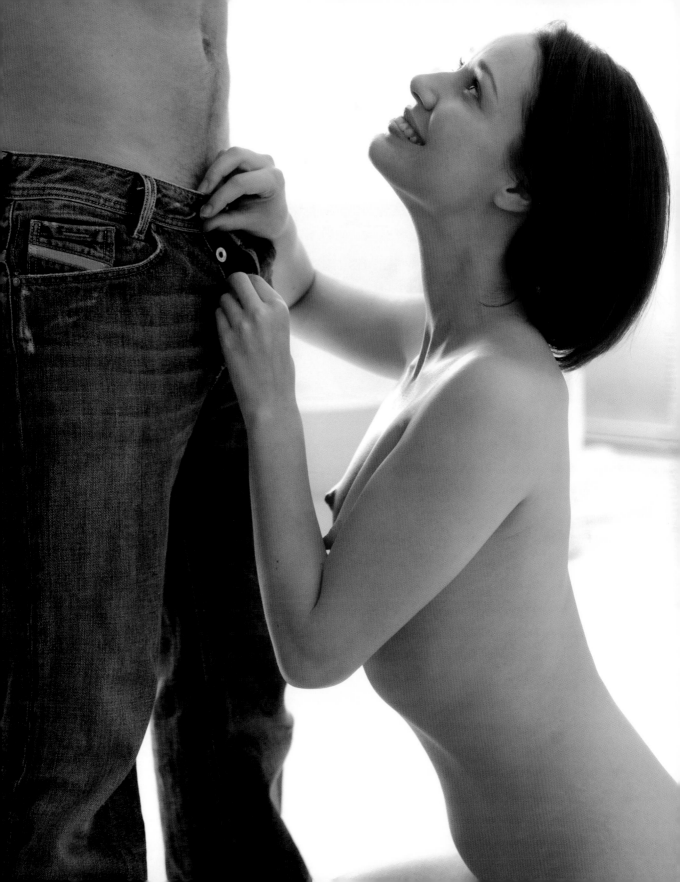

Cunnilingus

Cunnilingus is good for both of you—he has the thrill of delivering intense pleasure, while you get to lie back and abandon yourself to the moment. Plus you'll feel an intimate sexual bond that has the power to enhance your whole relationship. If you're used to giving pleasure rather than receiving it, cunnilingus may give you a rare opportunity to concentrate exclusively on yourself. You may find this sort of "selfishness" a challenge—but one that's definitely worth rising to.

Relax and accept yourself

A key part of enjoying oral sex is being at home in your skin and accepting your body and your sexuality. If oral sex doesn't feature in your sex life, it may be because you've consciously or unconsciously signaled to your lover that you don't enjoy it. Perhaps you feel self-conscious about the appearance or taste of your genitals. Or perhaps you have tried oral sex a few times, but it has fallen by the wayside.

Whatever the case, it's important to realize that both of you could be missing out if you aren't giving it a try. If you're worried about your genital smell or taste, remind yourself that your smell can be a natural aphrodisiac. Regular bathing is all you need to keep yourself smelling sweet. And if you rush straight from the shower to the bedroom, your lover is more likely to taste the chemicals in your shower gel than the far-sexier taste of you.

Before you start

Enjoying intimate acts such as cunnilingus often means getting into the right headspace—if you're feeling tense or you haven't unwound from your day, you're unlikely to give yourself up to the experience. Do whatever you need to get into a relaxed and sexy mindset—whether it's reading an erotic story or flirting with your lover. You might find it helpful to get in the right mood with deep, calming breathing exercises or extended foreplay.

Positions please

To start, get into a position that will give you the most stimulation, and your partner the least amount of neck strain. Try lying back on the bed with your lover kneeling between your legs. Put some cushions under your buttocks to make your genitals more accessible. You could also try standing with your lover at your feet. Alternatively, sit on the edge of your bed, or a chair or sofa, and let your man kneel before you.

Hitting the spot

When your man hits the right spot, give him plenty of feedback through your body language (push up your pelvis or gyrate your hips). And don't be inhibited when it comes to making a noise—your moans, gasps, and sighs will act as a powerful incentive for your lover to keep that rhythm going. Treat oral sex as the perfect opportunity to release your sexual vixen.

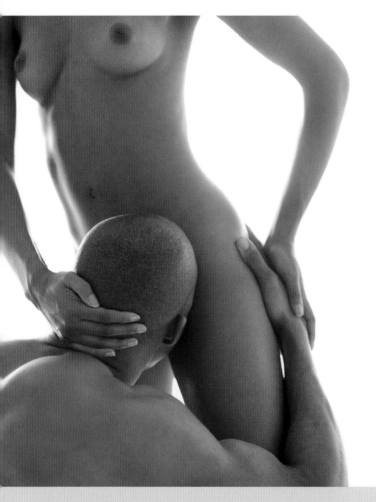

Take your time

Ask your man to start slowly by gently kissing your inner thighs and abdomen. Let him alternate between genital stimulation and caressing your breasts and nipples. This will heighten your response and leave you craving more. Have him kiss and gently lick around your labia and vagina. When you start to feel wet, ask him to open the lips with his fingers. Let him stimulate your clitoris and inside your vagina with his tongue. Ask him to use his fingers to stimulate your G-spot. Let him also kiss, suck, and lick your perineum.

Switching the pace

Let your man alternate between different speeds and pressures, avoiding random flicks and licks. Some men prefer to move their tongue in a figure-eight motion, while others find that spelling out the alphabet with their tongue works as well. Find the motion you prefer together, then let him tease you a little. He should keep his tongue well-lubricated so that the strokes are pleasurable for you. Revel in the sensations before he sends you over the edge.

The kiss of pleasure

Get your lover to place his mouth around your clitoris to create suction around the entire area, and let him use his tongue to delicately stimulate your clitoris. The varying sensations of being sucked and licked will give you intense pleasure. He can also try kissing and mouthing the peri-urethral area. This is very sensitive for you and will get you aroused and ready for more sex play.

Oral pleasure

Lie back, relax, and open up the most private part of your body to the delectable experience of being licked and sucked by your lover. Let him use his tongue to experiment and navigate his way to your clitoris, G-spot, and labia. With these three techniques to help him out, it won't be long before he's giving you the "kiss of pleasure."

Fellatio

Men love oral sex. The combination of your warm, wet mouth and lips and the texture of your tongue is enough to drive any man wild. Yet many couples find that oral sex falls by the wayside in their relationship and becomes something they do only on special occasions. This is not because women in long-term relationships regard oral sex as an activity belonging to their younger selves, but rather that when it's already hard to find time for a quickie, oral sex seems to be a luxury.

Intimate oral

It is easy to see how fellatio is something for special occasions, but engaging in it regularly is a sure way of keeping your relationship sexy and fresh. Performing fellatio on your man creates an instant and very intimate bond between the two of you. Oral sex demonstrates trust, love, and seductive power, while also telling your man that you think he is hot, and his genitals are sexy—vital to his self-esteem and body image. Plus, most men adore fellatio—even more, rumor has it, than "normal sex."

You may be worried about oral techniques, but with a few clever skills (and a wet tongue), it's easy to give your man good head. In fact, most men would agree that there is no such thing as bad oral sex. What's more, you don't need any special accessories to enjoy it—you don't even need to get undressed, making it great for a quickie. When you have more time, make oral sex part of foreplay to enhance your lovemaking sessions.

Positive approach

The spirit in which you give fellatio is as important as the techniques you use—more so, in fact. Fellatio that feels grudging or half-hearted won't

be pleasurable for either of you. So don't wait for him to ask—offer, or just unbuckle his belt with a look of sexy intent. And once you're down there, throw yourself into the action. Fellatio can be a great way to feel emotionally connected to your lover if you give yourself up to the experience. If you have reservations about fellatio being "dirty," concentrate on all the pleasurable aspects, such as the thrill of taking charge and being personally responsible for such intense pleasure.

Get comfortable

There are lots of sexy positions for giving fellatio. Try out a few different ones until you find one that gives you the least amount of neck strain.

The classic position is to have your partner lie on the bed while you kneel or lie over him and pleasure him. However, you might find it's more comfortable to kneel on a pillow between your partner's knees while he sits on the edge of a chair, the bed, or the sofa. All of these positions allow you to control the action. If you are a bit more daring, let him stand while you kneel in front. In this position, he will have more freedom to move and might not be able to resist giving the occasional thrust, so it's not for the uninitiated.

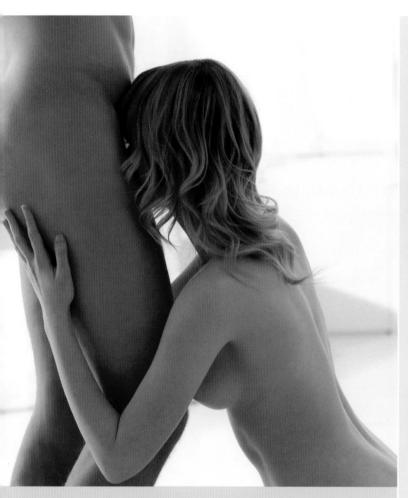

The big "O"

One of the most popular oral sex moves actually involves a lot of hand action. Place your hand over your mouth in an "O" shape. Take his penis in your mouth while keeping your hand over your mouth. As you move up and down the length of his shaft, use your hand to maintain pressure across the penis. You can also try twisting your hand gently across it as your mouth continues in an up-and-down motion. The result will be constant and varied sensations all over his penis—sure to blow his mind.

Simple oral pleasures

If you want to make a performance out of fellatio, turn on the lights and get your red lipstick out. Start by sensually applying color to your lips before turning your attention to his penis. A drink of water or warm herbal tea can keep your mouth moist, and a good lip balm will give a smooth slip to your lips. Sucking on a strong peppermint before giving head will give him wonderfully warm sensations as you suck him. Watching his penis moving in and out of your hot, red lips will give him an utterly orgasmic experience.

Good vibrations

Try humming during your oral session. The sensations created by your mouth and lips will create wonderful vibrations on your man's penis, and it can be a fun way to spice up a regular oral session. You don't have to hum a whole tune throughout—just vary different pitches and lengths while your mouth is on his penis. He can try this technique on you, too.

Oral delights

The basic oral sex moves are simple, and few sensations can match the feeling of your lips sliding down his shaft. But when you want to vary your moves, try these three suggestions. Adding a helping hand can be just what he needs to trigger his orgasm. So, too, can a pair of crimson lips, or some subtle vibrations that travel the length of his penis.

Sex files: Letting go of hang-ups

Sexual hang-ups prevent us from feeling free to give and receive pleasure in bed. If you're inhibited about things such as being naked or having sex in a particular position, your sex life can start to feel restricted or predictable. Here's how one woman overcame her ingrained resistance to oral sex.

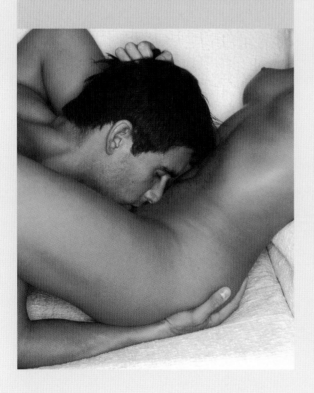

Background
Marc, 28, and Jasmine, 25, dated happily for 10 months before he asked her to marry him. They are looking forward to their wedding, and their relationship is close, loving, and committed.

The problem
Marc was worried about one aspect of his sex life with Jasmine—she didn't like giving or receiving oral sex. She'd do it to Mark if he begged her, or if she'd had a few drinks, but she'd never let him reciprocate. Marc said it wasn't just the lack of pleasure he was worried about, but the lack of trust and intimacy he sensed from Jasmine.

Jasmine said she simply didn't enjoy oral sex: "It's the only sexual thing I don't like. It's just a personal thing, like preferring chocolate ice cream to vanilla."

Finding solutions
Although I didn't want Jasmine to feel pressured, I asked her what, specifically, she found unappealing about oral sex. "Everything—the smell, the taste... I don't want anyone that close to me down there, and I don't feel happy being that close to someone else. Oral sex makes me feel dirty."

After reassuring her that these feelings were normal, we talked about Jasmine's adolescence. Despite being raised in a strict religious household, Jasmine said that she had been a "bad" teenager. She lost her virginity at 13 and had a reputation for being promiscuous.

When she left home to go to college she tried to reinvent herself as a "good girl." Although she felt she had succeeded in this, she still feels guilty about her past, and is eager to distance herself from anything she considers "dirty." Jasmine also said she was ashamed of her genitals and referred to them only as "down there."

To encourage Jasmine to be more comfortable with her sexuality, I asked her to write a list of all the things she liked about sex with Marc. We also discussed how negative messages about sex from our parents can lead to guilt, inhibitions, and sexual shame. Jasmine agreed that she'd been taught that "nice girls don't have sex," but that she wanted to let go of that belief.

As part of her homework I asked Jasmine to become more informed about her genital anatomy and to look at her genitals in a handheld mirror. I hoped, in time, Jasmine would find the idea of Marc being close to her genitals less shocking and uncomfortable.

I recommended to Marc that he should take the issue of oral sex off the table for the moment. Rather than bringing it up every time they were intimate, I suggested that Marc let Jasmine lead the way. I felt that once Marc and Jasmine were married, Jasmine's inhibitions in the bedroom would slowly start to resolve themselves.

I also asked Marc to compliment Jasmine's genitals to make her less insecure about their appearance and odor. And I suggested that he compliment her sexual technique overall to boost her confidence.

What happened?

Within a few months Jasmine became more sexually adventurous and open to the idea of giving and receiving oral sex, although it's still not one of her favorite activities. Marc is happier with their sex life and is now content to let Jasmine take the lead.

Find a compromise

If you have a sexual hang-up, avoid "banning" a particular act or position. Instead, talk to your partner to see if you can reach a compromise. And work at challenging and overcoming inhibitions—this will help you and your relationship to grow, both in and out of bed.

Tried-and-tested positions

Some of the best positions are the ones that are most commonly used. They are comfortable and pleasurable for both partners, and are accessible to most couples. What makes these positions so beloved? They give you intimacy, a fantastic sensory experience, and reliably fulfilling sex—perfect for days when all you want is the moves that work. Far from being mundane, with a few variations (and a couple of pillows), you can bring some fireworks to these everyday greats.

Classics that work

The missionary position is famous for good reason. It feels great for your man, because he gets to control the action, and it involves the least amount of energy on your part—ideal when you don't feel like a workout. Woman-on-top is another classic favorite with couples for similar, but opposing, reasons. You work up a sweat doing it but get to control the thrust and depth of penetration. Your man gets to watch you take charge while enjoying a good time.

Both of these positions promise relationship-enhancing sex. They put you face to face with your lover, so you can kiss, nuzzle, and caress your way to the perfect orgasm. Give each other eye contact and you will enjoy a unique, and very sexy, bonding experience with your lover.

For a slight change of pace, try sitting sideways to access a different angle of penetration. Alternatively, standing and man-from-behind positions feel a bit naughty.

Refining your technique

How can you get the most out of these positions? First, be aware of what you want from a sexual move—more or less control, deep penetration,

shallow thrusts, or G-spot stimulation, for example. This is important in determining the types of position that work best for you and your partner. Only the first third of your vagina is highly sensitive, so the deep thrusts that accompany missionary-style positions may not be stimulating the most sensitive parts of your vagina. If this is the case, ask your partner to alternate shallow thrusts—in which he almost exits your vagina—with deep thrusts to heighten your pleasure (and also prevent him from climaxing too quickly).

Enhancing the everyday

Even when your sex life is utterly fulfilling, it's great to take your favorite positions to the next level by adding a few props. Handcuffs or other light restraints are perfect for light-hearted sexual games of domination and submission.

You could also add an element of fantasy. Ask him to tie your arms loosely with a silk scarf, and act out a scenario in which he is taking you against your will. Alternatively he could blindfold you and take control of your senses. This will lead you to experience heightened anticipation and sensory perception—you won't know where his hands or lips will travel next.

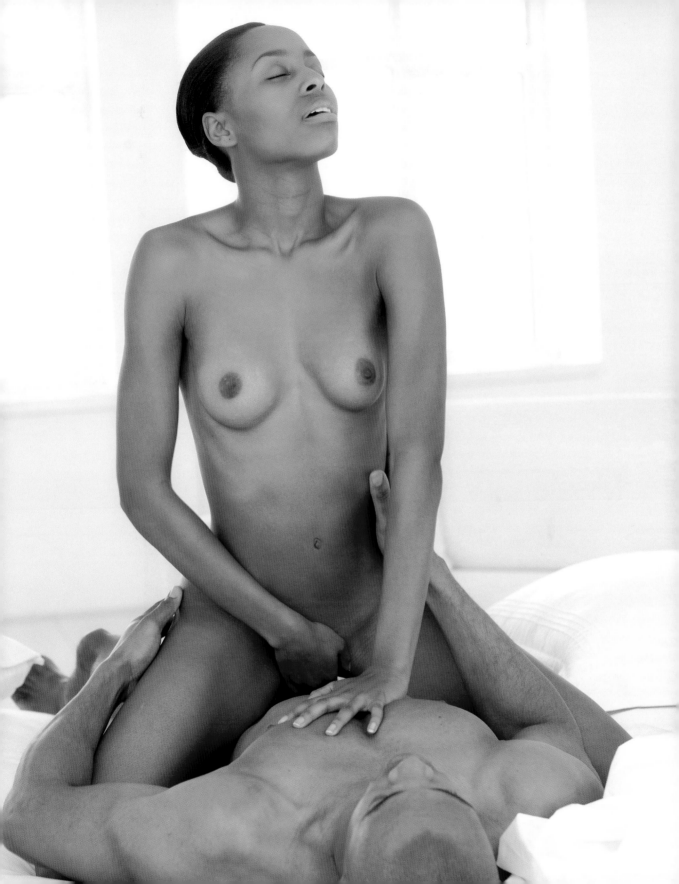

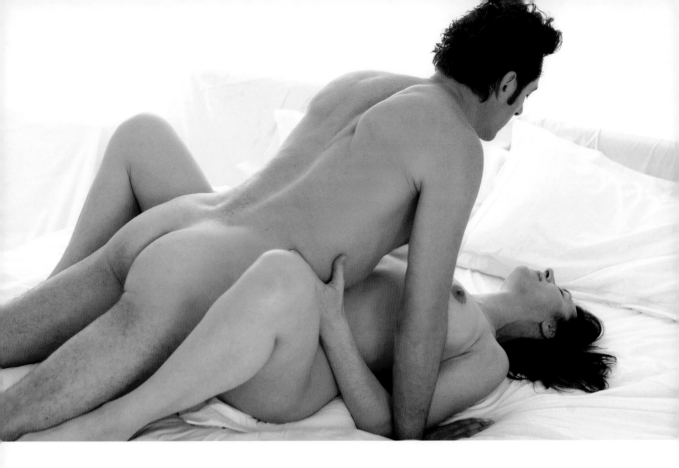

Missionary

Close positions such as the missionary allow for very intimate lovemaking. Use the opportunity to kiss, nibble, nuzzle, and whisper sexy thoughts to each other. You will enjoy the sensations of his deep thrusts, while he will love being able to watch your every reaction. The most instinctive lovemaking position, the classic missionary allows you to experiment with new ways of touching, kissing, and pleasuring each other during sex. It also allows you to watch each other reach orgasm. Don't be afraid of the "orgasm face." It is a special connection between you and your partner, and the missionary and all its variations are excellent for reveling in this private, erotic part of your relationship.

Classic missionary position

◄ For maximum intimacy, the classic missionary can't be beat. Face-to-face action lets you open up to each other in a very erotic way.

Leg action

▶ A bit of leg action can add a little kinky pleasure to the standard missionary. Lie back and bend your legs in the air. Your man kneels before you and rests your legs against his shoulders. From this position, he will be able to thrust deeply into you. Drawing your legs up toward him will move your pelvis up and down on his penis. Alternately, he can hold your legs upright against your chest. He will enjoy the sense of control while watching the pleasure on your face, and you will experience increased stimulation of your clitoris and cervix. He can combine his deeper thrusts with shallower ones to stimulate your G-spot as well.

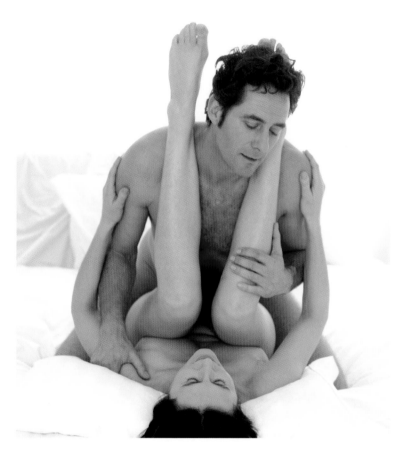

Bee's knees

▶ For the more athletically inclined, this position will help your man get even deeper into you. Lie flat on your back with one of your ankles resting on his shoulder, and your other knee bent. Have your man get into a half-lying/half-kneeling position on top of you. Use your thighs for leverage as you rock back and forth together. This action will tighten your vagina around his penis. You can also stimulate your clitoris with your hand as he thrusts. Lifting both of your legs in the air gives him a tighter position, resulting in heightened sensations on your clitoris.

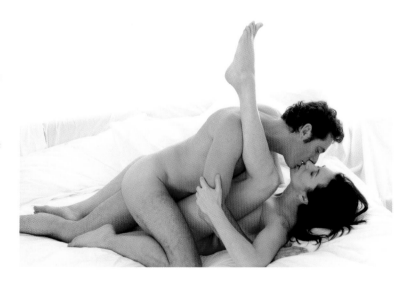

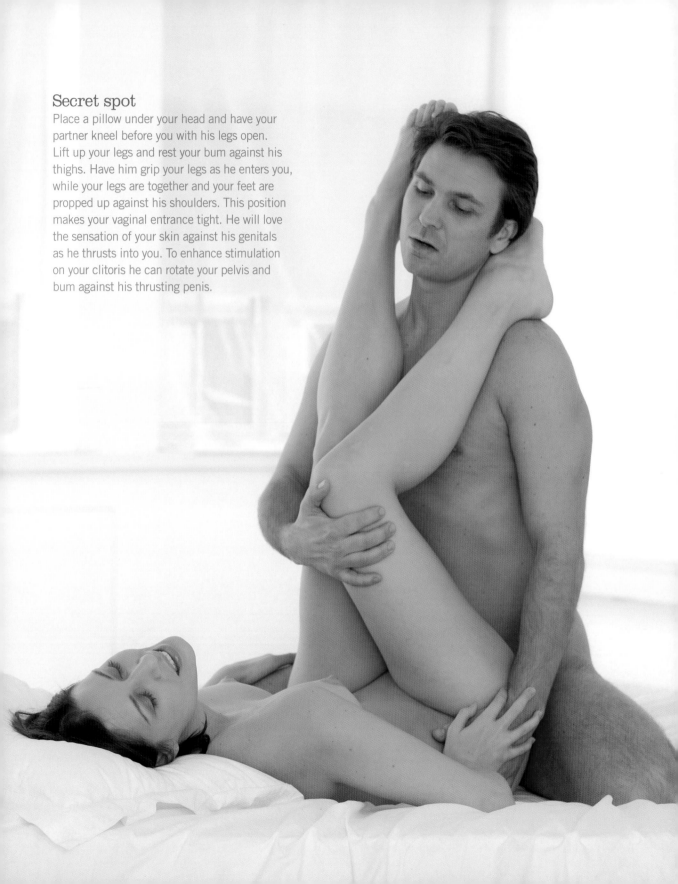

Secret spot

Place a pillow under your head and have your partner kneel before you with his legs open. Lift up your legs and rest your bum against his thighs. Have him grip your legs as he enters you, while your legs are together and your feet are propped up against his shoulders. This position makes your vaginal entrance tight. He will love the sensation of your skin against his genitals as he thrusts into you. To enhance stimulation on your clitoris he can rotate your pelvis and bum against his thrusting penis.

V-shape

▶ Lie on your back with your legs in the air in the shape of a "V." Your partner should kneel between your legs to enter you. From this position he will have the freedom to thrust deeply. Enjoy the penetration as you move your pelvis up and down on his penis in rhythm with his movements. Your G-spot will receive added pressure and massage from his penis. For extra stimulation, caress his genitals or your clitoris.

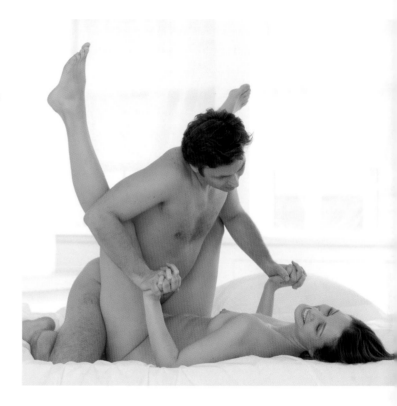

Pillow partners

▼ This intimate position means you can lie back and make flirty eye contact with each other. Relax on the bed and raise your pelvis with some pillows. Keep your knees slightly bent and your feet flat on the floor or bed. Your man should position himself between your knees and support himself on his arms. Now he can penetrate you deeply, while you rock in sync with his thrusting. Arch your back to allow him to penetrate you deeply.

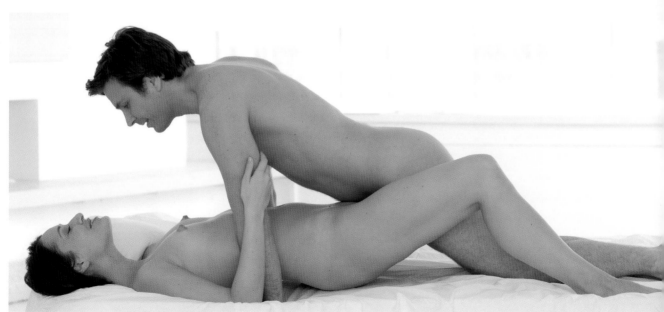

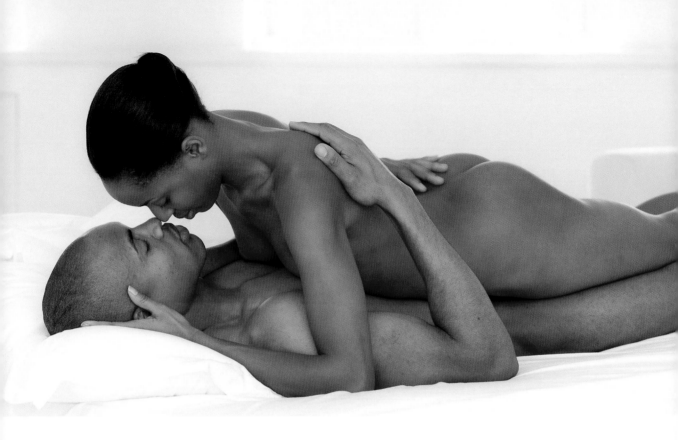

Woman on top

This "daring diva" position has been popularized in sexology for centuries and fantasized about by most men. In woman-on-top positions, the woman straddles her partner and then determines the depth and rhythm of intercourse. You can kiss, caress, and stroke each other to orgasm. If you feel self-conscious about having your body on full display, never fear—this show is what men absolutely love about having sex. It means they get to lie back, get a full view of you, and let you do all the hard work. Meanwhile, enjoy being able to control the pace and thrust of sex. You get to determine what happens, and he will be able to caress and stroke your breasts, back, and bottom. What more can you ask for?

Flat face-to-face

◀ This intimate position allows you to gaze into each other's eyes, embrace tenderly, and feel maximum body-to-body contact along the length of your bodies, with your legs aligned.

Deep down

▶ In this seated woman-on-top position, you will enjoy complete control and experience deep penetration. You will probably find that the head of his penis touches or stimulates your cervix, so make sure you are fully aroused before trying this one. Sit down on his penis with your knees bent and your feet under or next to his arms. Place your hands behind you and grip his legs for balance. You will both enjoy the sensation of intense pressure on your genitals as you rock back and forth. One caveat: Be careful not to lean back too far, or you risk bending his penis, which is very painful.

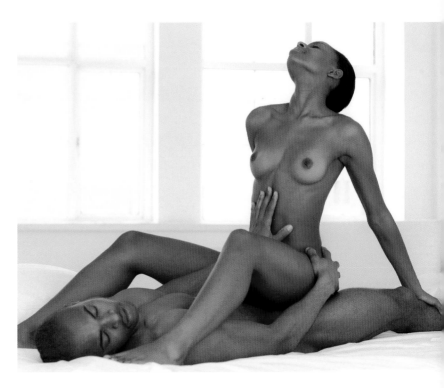

Kneel-'n'-straddle

▶ This kneeling position allows you all the comfort and control of kneeling, but it also heightens your man's excitement since he gets to be up close and personal with your behind. Ask your partner to lie on his back with one knee bent, then kneel astride him facing his feet. Your back should arch away from his bent knee. By rubbing your groin against his leg, you will stimulate your clitoris. Rest your hand on his chest for support, and use his leg for balance as you grind up and down on his penis.

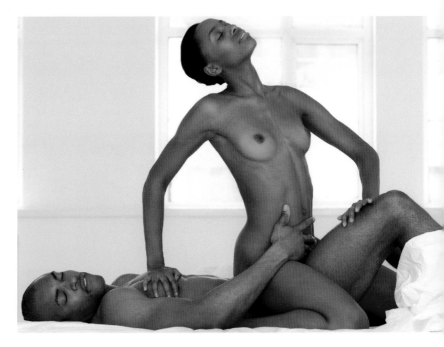

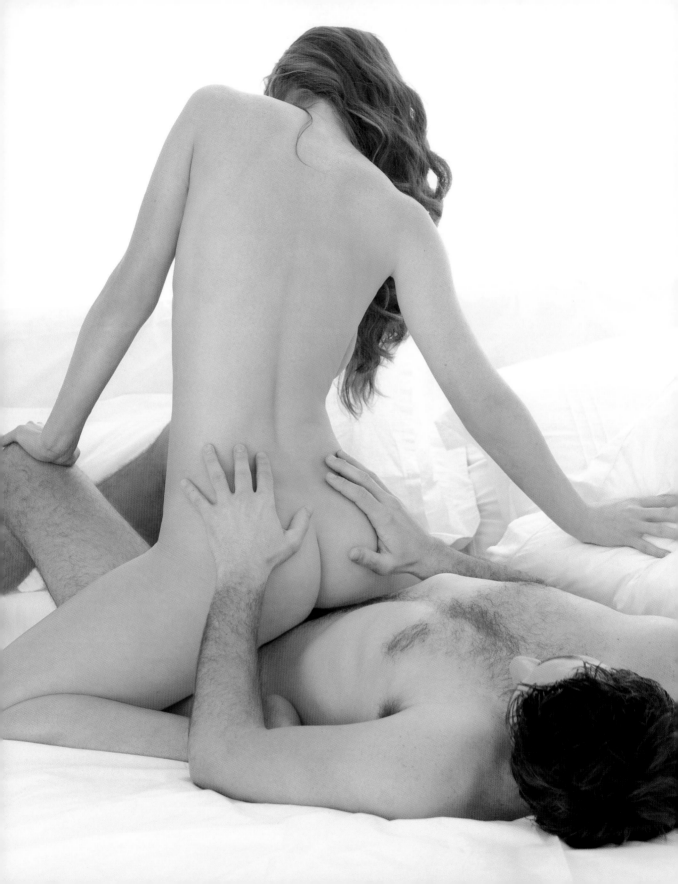

Rear assets

◄ With your man's knees bent and his legs spread, kneel astride him and lower yourself onto his penis. Don't put all your weight on him. For his comfort and yours, maintain some of your weight in your legs by keeping your knees bent and your legs taut. You now have the power of a woman-on-top position combined with a doggy-style view for his pleasure— the perfect position for both of you.

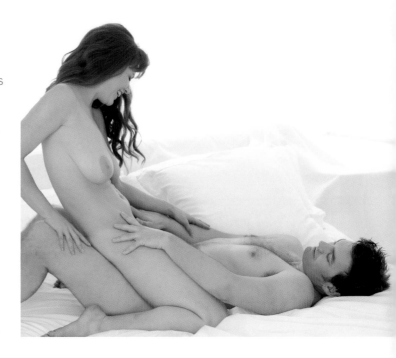

Figure-eight

▶ This is a breathtakingly easy and orgasmic position for you, because it puts you in complete control of the thrust and angle of penetration. Your man lies flat on his back with his knees bent before him. You sit astride him on your knees, and lean back against his thighs. Sit comfortably on his penis, then gyrate your hips, grind back and forth, or swirl your pelvis in a sexy figure-eight motion. Use this sexy technique whenever you are on top to slow things down and inject an added sense of playfulness into your lovemaking.

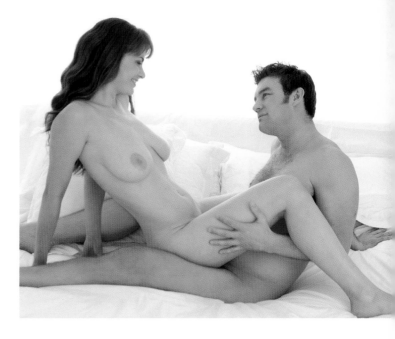

Eye-to-eye

▶ Lean back on your arms and enjoy an intimate lovemaking session gazing into your lover's eyes. Your man should sit with his legs slightly bent before him and one arm behind. Seat yourself comfortably between his legs, with your legs behind him on either side. Your partner can use his free hand to caress your thigh or your breasts, or to stimulate your clitoris. In return, you will be able to rock and rub your lover to a divinely close climax.

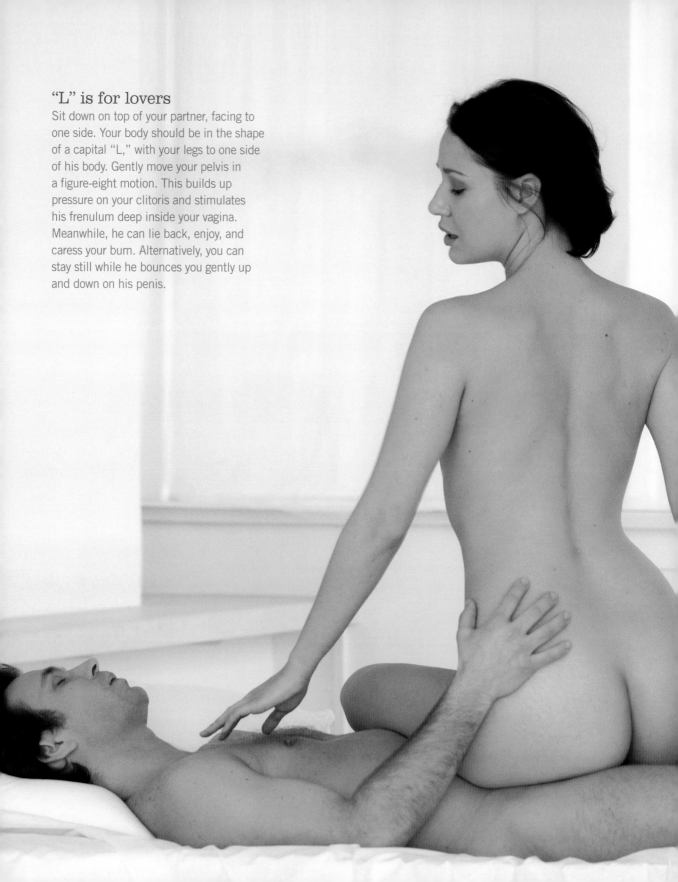

"L" is for lovers

Sit down on top of your partner, facing to
one side. Your body should be in the shape
of a capital "L," with your legs to one side
of his body. Gently move your pelvis in
a figure-eight motion. This builds up
pressure on your clitoris and stimulates
his frenulum deep inside your vagina.
Meanwhile, he can lie back, enjoy, and
caress your bum. Alternatively, you can
stay still while he bounces you gently up
and down on his penis.

Merry go round

▶ For a different twist on woman on top, try doing a complete 180-degree turn. To get into position, lie on top of your man. His head should be at your feet and your feet at his head. You may need to straddle him and then slowly rotate. In this position, his penis will feel surprisingly different than it usually does. Use your muscles to squeeze it, then wriggle your pelvis to create different rhythms.

Top up

▼ Enjoy the control of being on top coupled with the comfort and ease of the missionary position. Have your man lean back on one arm, with his legs open in front of him. Sit down on top of him, then recline so that your legs are in front of you and behind him. Use a pillow under your shoulder for comfort. Lie back, enjoy, and clasp hands while he rocks back and forth inside of you.

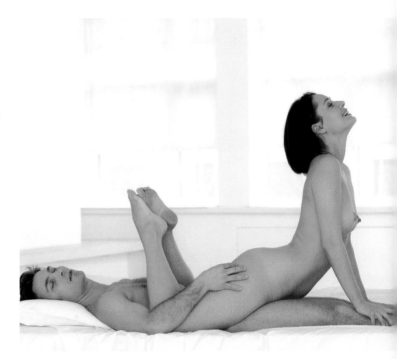

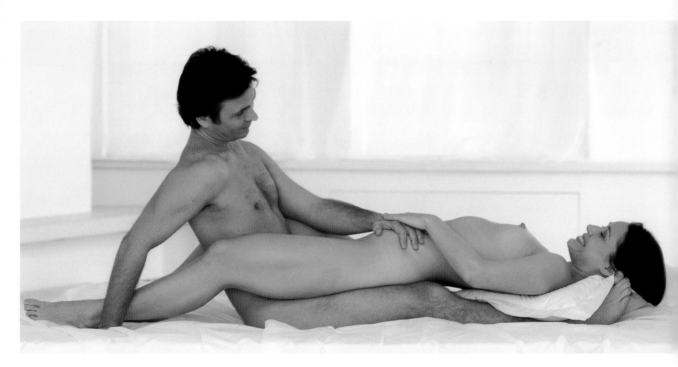

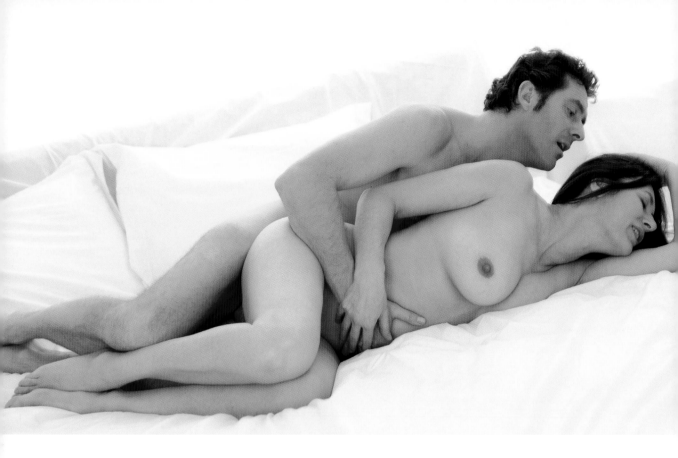

Sideways

The *Kama Sutra* recommends this position for newlyweds who are just learning about lovemaking, probably because it is an easy, comfortable position, which enhances intimacy and romance. Not only is the side-by-side position very bonding, it is perfect for those sleepy-time or just-woken-up, must-have-sex-now moments. If you are lying in the classic spoon position—with your body facing away from your partner—it is an excellent position for clitoral stimulation. Turn and lie face to face, and you can maintain eye contact with your lover and still receive clitoral pleasure from the friction between your bodies. Sideways positions also keep your vaginal entrance tight.

Sweet snuggle

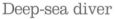 A perfect position for sleepy-time bonding or those early-morning encounters, all that spoon-shaped sex requires is an arched back from you and some gentle thrusts from him.

Top dog

▶ In this sexy position, your man will enjoy the excitement of a doggy-style position while you recline on your side. Spread your legs slightly to allow your partner to enter you. This will make your vagina feel tight. Your lover kneels or reclines behind you, allowing the friction from his penis to stimulate your clitoris. Enjoy watching your partner's body and face as you head toward climax. He can help you along by caressing your breasts and body. Enjoy the sense of intimacy and closeness that this position creates.

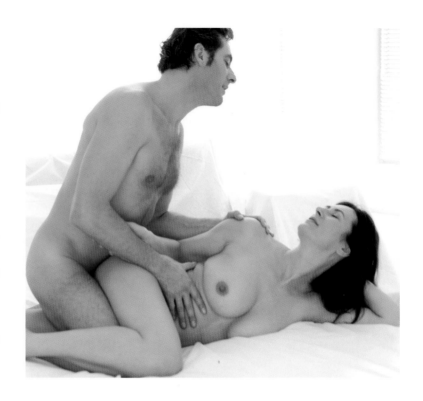

Deep-sea diver

▶ This is a restful position that also gives you deep vaginal penetration. To get into this sexy move, lie on your side with your head resting on your bent arm. Your man lies perpendicular to you, while turning sideways to enter you. In essence, he will be lying between your legs while using his pelvis to thrust deeply and stimulate your cervix. Shallower thrusts will build up pressure on your G-spot. He can place his arms on the bed or your back to help him balance. In this position, you can reach down to stimulate your clitoris. You can also reach between your legs to caress your man's inner thigh and gently massage his testicles and perineum— truly orgasmic.

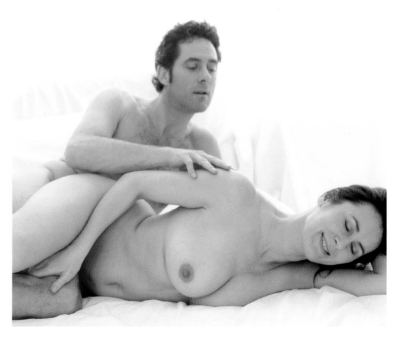

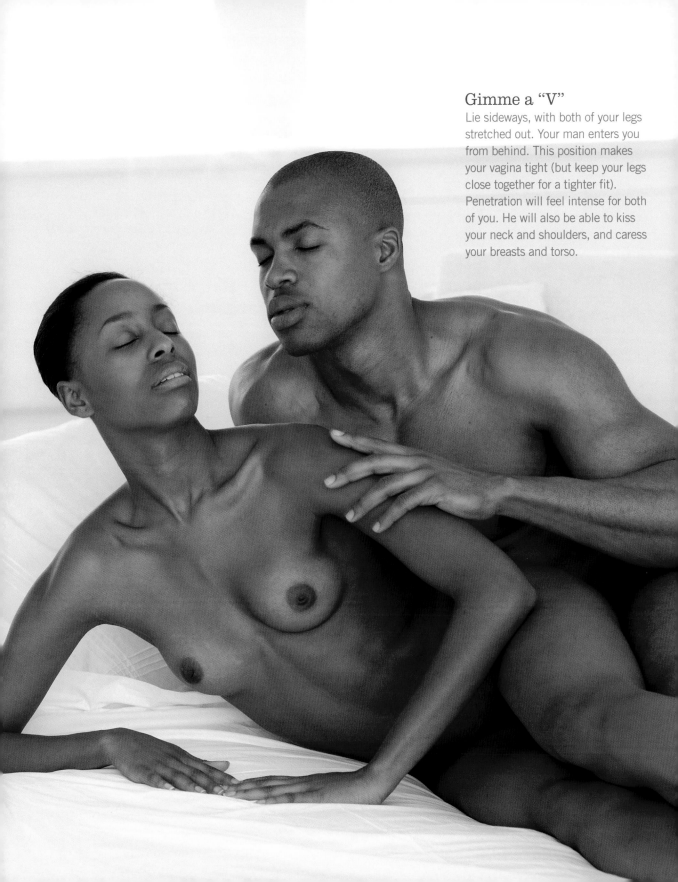

Gimme a "V"

Lie sideways, with both of your legs stretched out. Your man enters you from behind. This position makes your vagina tight (but keep your legs close together for a tighter fit). Penetration will feel intense for both of you. He will also be able to kiss your neck and shoulders, and caress your breasts and torso.

The wrap

▶ This is a position for when you want to snuggle up, kiss deeply, and enjoy being close. Lie on your sides, facing each other. His pelvis should be slightly angled in the direction he is facing. Wrap your arms and legs around his body, and slowly angle yourself onto his penis. Move your pelvis in tighter to enjoy deep penetration. The proximity of bodies will create friction on your clitoris, while you and your man can caress each other to climax.

Free bird

▼ In this sexy spoon, your man lies behind and you open your legs to let him enter you. Have him take your uppermost leg and pull it gently behind him (or hold it in the air). This tightens your vaginal muscles, increasing pressure on his penis and your hot spots. It may look tricky, but it is actually an easy and restful position to assume. Your partner can wrap his arm around you to create the warmth of spooning.

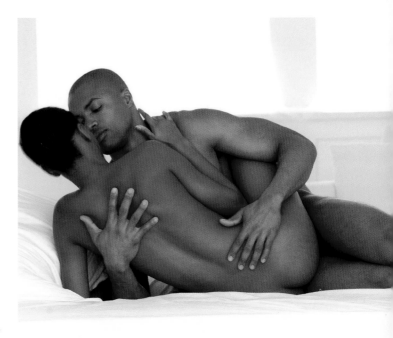

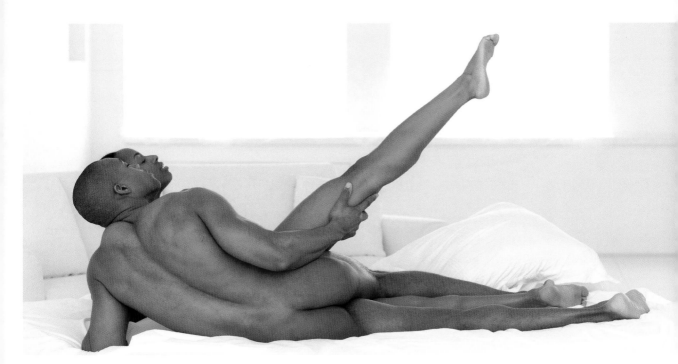

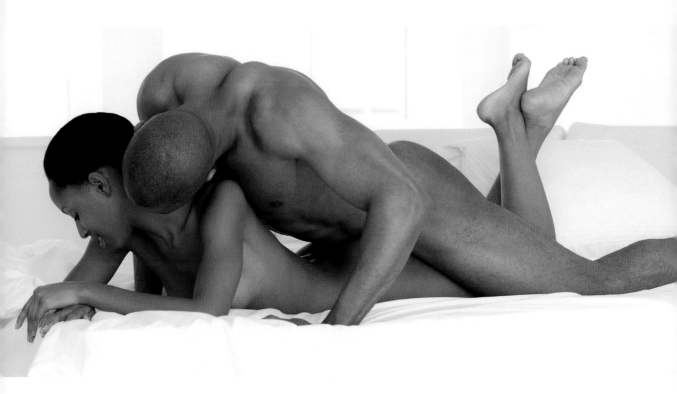

Doggy-style

Being penetrated from behind is the most animalistic of all positions. Doggy-style allows men and women to get in touch with their primal urges and express their sexuality. He will love watching his penis entering you, and you will love the stimulation he can offer with his free hands. Prop yourself up on your elbows for maximum G-spot stimulation, or try lying on your stomach. Double the pleasure for both of you and use your fingers to stimulate yourself while your man penetrates you, or just let the friction from the sheets create clitoral stimulation. The possibilities are endless. Just remember to wiggle, squirm, and swivel your hips as he thrusts from behind to enjoy a mind-blowing orgasm.

Lying-down dog
◀ Lie flat on your belly so that your man can lie over you, supporting his weight on his hands. Because your legs are close together, you will both feel very tightly connected—he will relish the compact fit of your vagina around his penis. Enjoy the deep penetration that this position allows—plus the erotic neck nibbles that he is ideally placed to give you.

Sitting spoons
▶ Ask your man to kneel on the bed. While facing away from him, lower yourself onto his penis. In this position, he can bounce you up and down while you rock back and forth. This builds pressure on his frenulum and your G-spot.

Crouching tiger
▼ This position is the ultimate in submissive and dominant pleasure. Place a pillow underneath your lower abdomen and prop yourself up on your elbows. Your partner can recline behind you, with his feet at each side and his arms supporting his weight behind him. From here, he can lay his bottom partially on your pillow and enter smoothly.

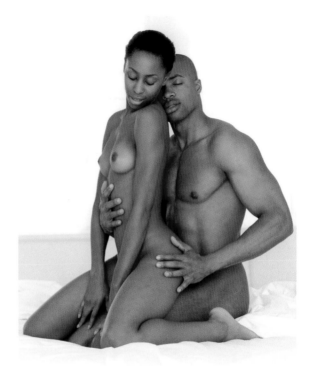

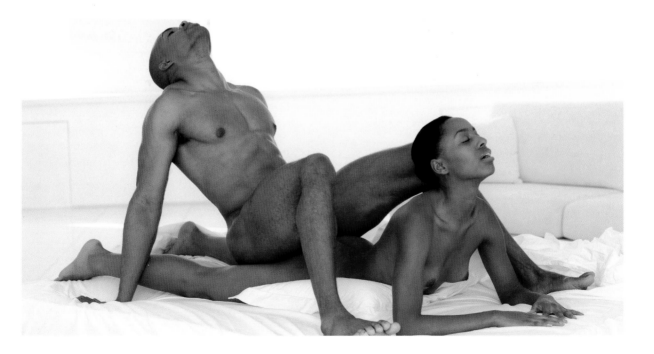

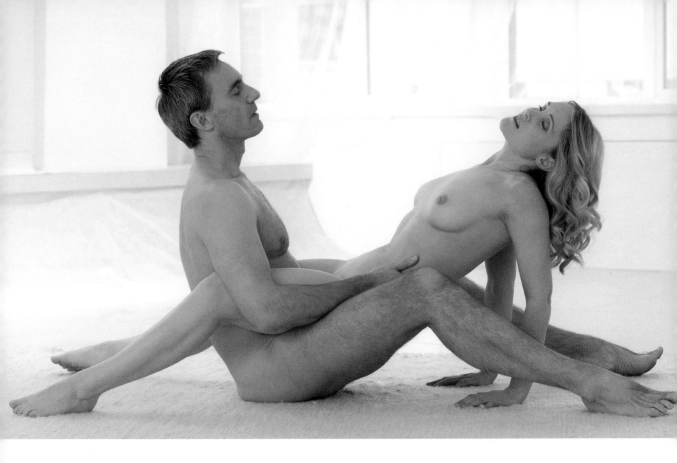

Sitting, kneeling, and standing

All of these positions will turn you on and are perfect for nonconventional sex—and combining one or two of them makes for an especially erotic lovemaking session. So when snuggling and kissing in front of the TV turns to naked passion, don't let going to bed break the spell and spoil the moment. Have sex right where you are, sitting or kneeling on the living room floor. If you make it to the bedroom, the bounce of the mattress works with sitting positions to create mind-blowing friction. You will be on top, so let your inner vixen come out and play. Making love standing up is for those times when you have to have each other now—on the stairs, against a doorway, near the kitchen counter: see where lust leads.

Friday-night sex

◀ This is a great position for nights when there's nothing on TV. Your partner sits on the floor with his legs bent and feet flat on the floor. Sit on his lap and lean back on your arms while he helps support your weight. You can place your feet on the floor or raise them akimbo to vary your clitoral sensations. This is a great position to show off your body and let him admire you.

Sexy back

▶ Stray from traditional in-and-out sex by sitting on your man's lap facing him. Wrap your arms around each other and enjoy kissing and staring into each other's eyes, while you gyrate and rock back and forth on his penis. This position is great for intimate, any-time sex.

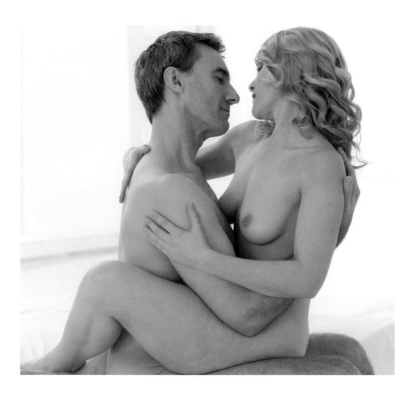

Sitting pretty

▶ This classic position is very relaxing. Your man will love the view, while being able to caress your gyrating bottom. He can sit on a chair or, if he prefers, recline on the bed or a sofa. As you face away from him, lower yourself provocatively onto his penis. In this position, you can place your arms on either side of him for support, or lean forward and grip his knees. Your man can reach round and caress your breasts or your clitoris from this position. This is a great little move for stimulating your clitoris while putting you in control of the depth and speed of penetration. Your lover will enjoy all the different sensations you create as you rock, wiggle, and move up and down.

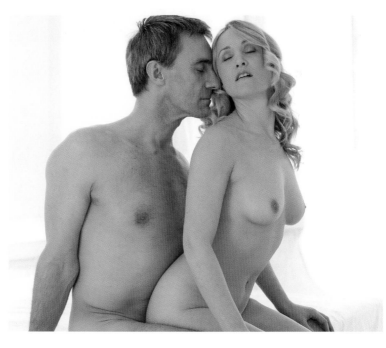

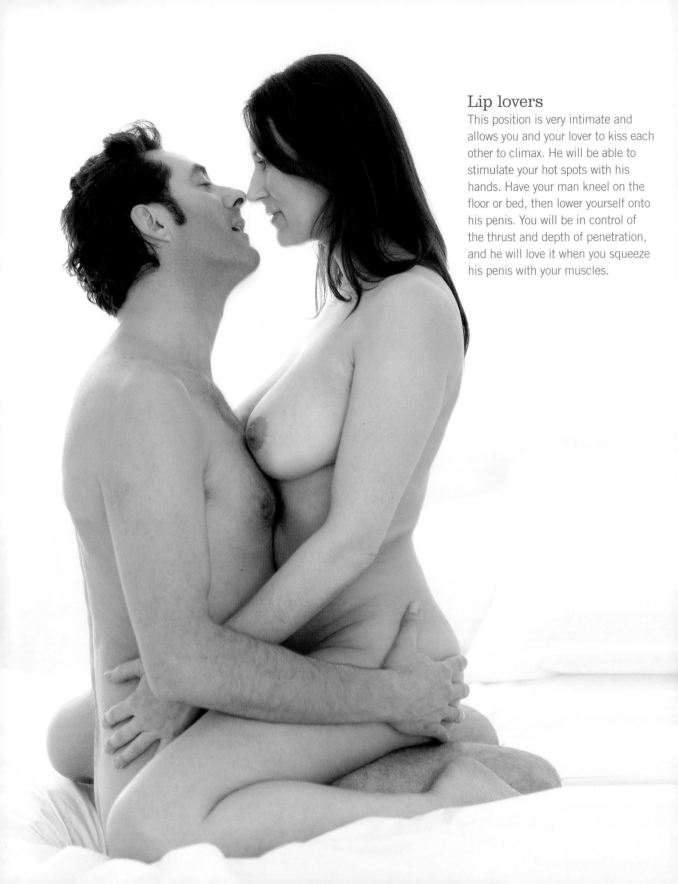

Lip lovers

This position is very intimate and allows you and your lover to kiss each other to climax. He will be able to stimulate your hot spots with his hands. Have your man kneel on the floor or bed, then lower yourself onto his penis. You will be in control of the thrust and depth of penetration, and he will love it when you squeeze his penis with your muscles.

Bottoms up

▶ This one is good for when you're feeling tired and he wants a quickie—you don't even need to remove all your clothes to get the moves. Kneel on the floor and lean your head on your hands and stick your bottom out. From this position, he can kneel and enter you from behind. Arch your back to experience deeper penetration. He will love being able to kiss other areas of your body while controlling the pace of sex. Add a little bounce by doing it on the bed—it will stop you from getting rug burn on your knees, and you will have more freedom to bounce and jiggle.

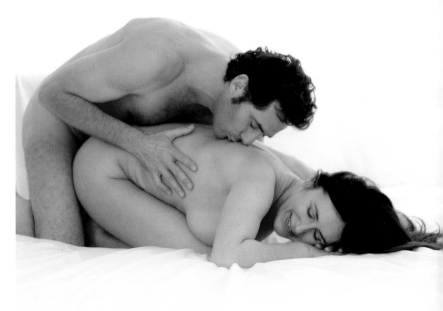

Lovers' lock

▶ Your man should sit with his legs crossed on the floor and lean back, supporting himself on his arms. Gently lower yourself down on his penis so that you are straddling it in a kneeling position. His penis will be in the perfect position to deeply penetrate you and stimulate your clitoris. Using his shoulders for support, make figure-eight motions with your pelvis. Great for enjoying uninhibited sex, this position gives you complete control as you rock back and forth on his penis. Neither of you will last very long with such intimate sensations. If your man has a thing for your bottom and you want G-spot stimulation, simply turn around to face the other direction.

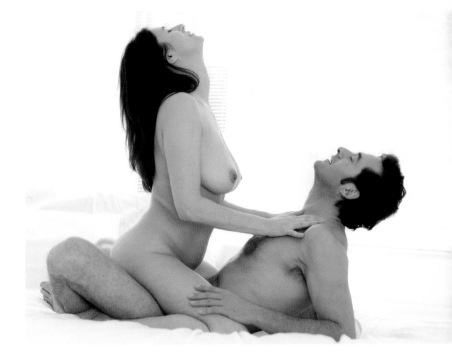

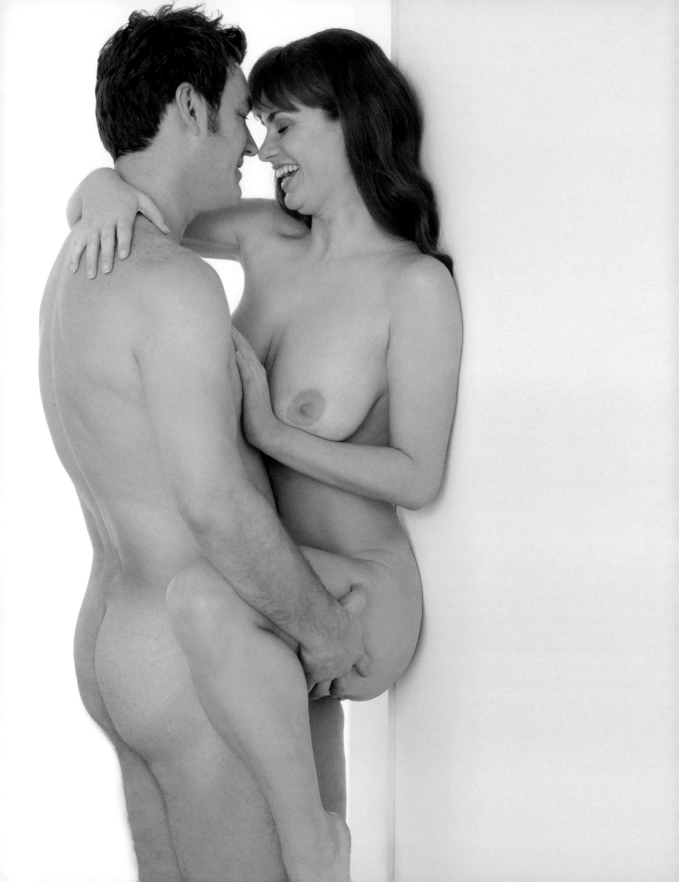

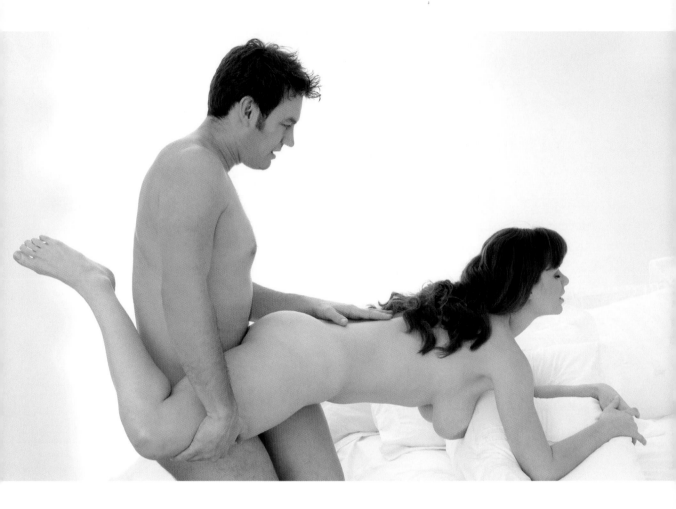

Against the wall

◄ This sexy and intimate pose is best for when you are craving a really intimate moment. As your man presses you against the wall, wrap your arms and one of your legs around him, then hold on tightly. With his hands under your bottom, he can keep you stable while entering you. He can also use this hand to stroke your labia and stimulate your clitoris. When he is getting close to orgasm, reach down and gently cup his testicles with your hand, or reach behind him to massage and stimulate his anal area. A variation on this position is to turn and lean against the wall as he enters you from behind.

Push up

▲ This position looks impressive but is actually quite easy to achieve, because you use your hands to help you balance. It also gives him plenty of room to penetrate, and he will enjoy being able to control the thrust and rhythm of your lovemaking. To get into this daring little number, you lean over the bed. He stands behind and lifts one of your legs, while you balance on your palms and elbows, either on the floor or on the bed. To take this position to the next level—and to let your man take complete control of your pleasure—he can lift both your legs, as though pushing a wheelbarrow.

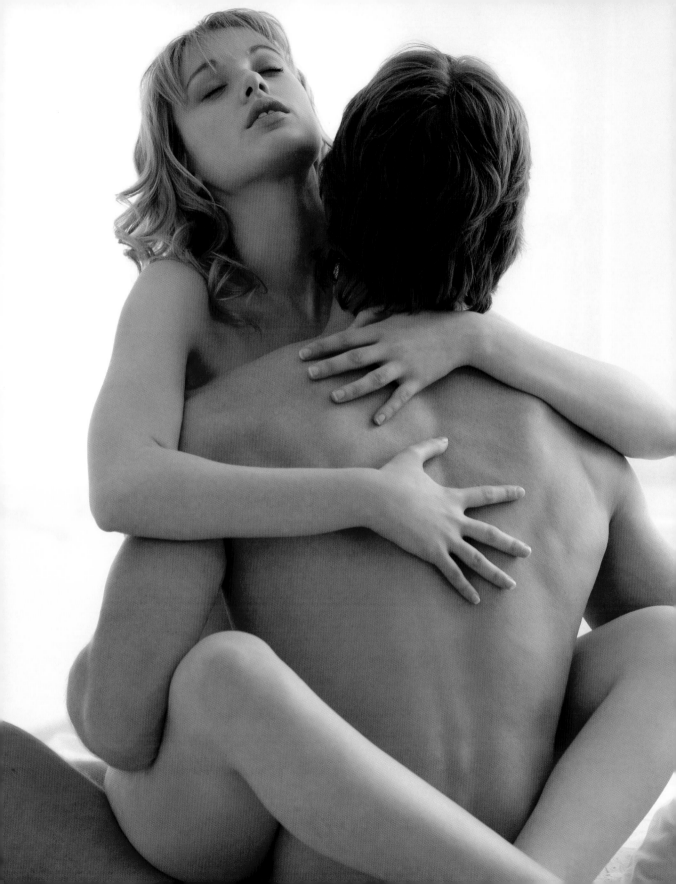

Sex reinvented

It's time to get creative now. Try out the techniques in this chapter and you'll find it's easy to unleash your inner sex goddess. Extend your boundaries with a sex toy, explore the world of erotica, or have an adrenalin-boosting adventure in a new location. Experiment with Coital Alignment Technique (CAT) for an orgasmic evening, or connect to the spiritual side of sex with Tantric lovemaking. All in all, get out of your comfort zone and enjoy some different moves. You'll find new stimulation, intimacy, and, above all, breathtaking orgasms.

Trying something new

Implementing something new in the bedroom requires a little bravery. From positions that put us face to face with body-image issues to sex that makes us slow down, breathe, and concentrate, braving the unknown in the bedroom can feel a little overwhelming, but it can also be amazingly erotic. Sex is not just about orgasm, it's about your connection with another sexual being. New positions, new techniques, and new sensations will enhance intimacy between you and keep your sex life hot.

A renewed sex life

Why not just keep practicing the same old moves? In order to enjoy the fullness of the beauty of sex, we have to shed our usual habits and be willing to experience sex with all of our senses engaged and all of our inhibitions quieted.

Learning about sex is a lifelong process, which some believe to be a spiritual quest. In the *Kama Sutra*, sex is respected as part of the beauty of life. Meditative, or spiritual, sex is found in the traditional arts of Tantric lovemaking. By practicing Tantric breathing, stroking, and gazing you can connect with your lover both spiritually and emotionally–vital for maintaining a good partnership over an extended time.

When you release your sexuality and use your body to give and receive pleasure, you will build a stronger sex life and day-to-day relationship. The only problem: you may never be satisfied with making love in missionary with the lights off again!

New positions

Fresh positions for sex allow you to experience new sensations. Positions such as Coital Alignment Technique (CAT), in which you and your lover rock your way to an amazing orgasm, or V-neck, where your man uses his penis to stimulate your clitoris, can provide novelty and intensity. Anal sex feels naughty, but enhances intimacy in your relationship and teaches you how to extend pleasure boundaries.

New techniques

You can improve nearly all positions with a few erotic tools. Take your pick from blindfolds, sex toys, and feathers. Use pillows to prop up your pelvis, cushion your bum or your knees, and change the angle of penetration for a whole new sex experience. Use chairs to improve some positions, particularly doggy-style. Vibrators, or a cock ring for him, can heighten orgasmic pleasure for both of you. If you are feeling adventurous, use props, accessories, and toys to enhance oral sex, too.

New locations

Move out of the bedroom and try the shower, the kitchen counter, or a night under the stars to add an adrenalin boost to your sex life. New locations usually mean new positions because there are no covers to hide under. So try leaning against a wall, over an office desk, or sitting on a swing seat.

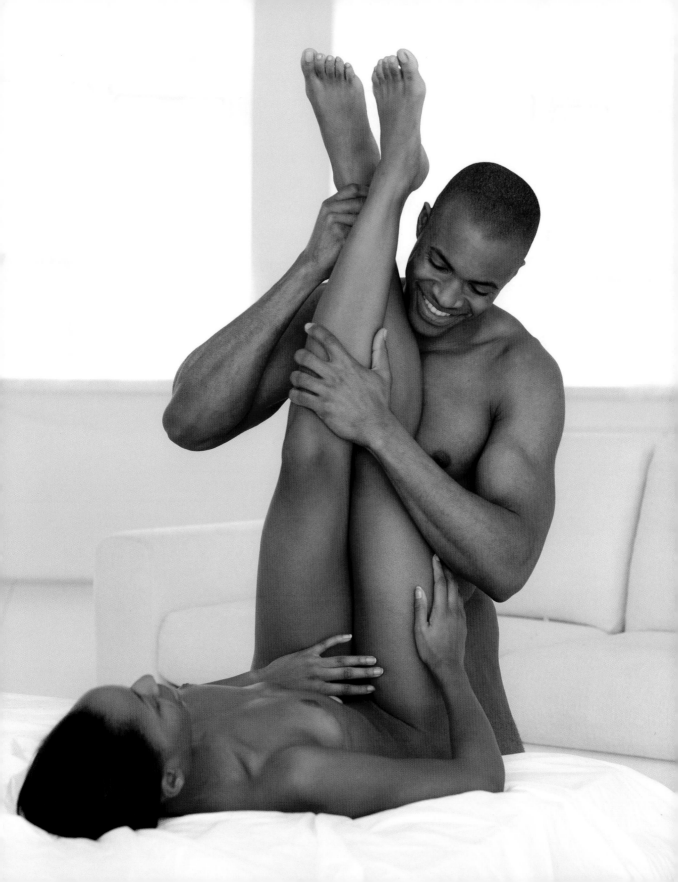

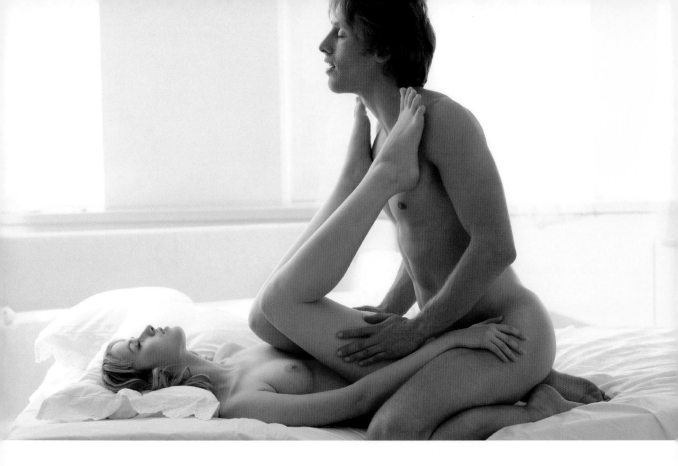

Orgasm-enhancing positions

Many couples delve into the *Kama Sutra* in search of orgasmic sex moves. These are not just about getting your body into the "correct" position; they also require you and your partner to be willing to open up your body to new sensations and to engage all of your senses. When that happens, these positions are especially likely to help you achieve orgasms that you will remember for weeks, months—maybe years to come. The most orgasm-friendly positions are those that allow for manual clitoral stimulation, and those that create pressure on the G-spot. Some of these moves can even lead to female ejaculation—a sight that's sure to make your partner request a return to these positions again and again.

Rising missionary

◀ This is the perfect position to achieve deeper intimacy and prime you both to reach mutual orgasm. Lie on your back and place your feet against your partner's shoulders. Let him kneel in front of you so that he can enter you deeply. This is a very intimate position that allows your man to see your face while he strokes your thighs, rubs your clitoris, and stimulates your anal region. He can control the depth and speed of his thrusts, but you will still have the freedom to move your pelvis up and down or in figure-eight motions. He can change his rhythm and can tease you by almost pulling out and then thrusting deeply again. This will also build up pressure on your G-spot, while you lie back and concentrate on having all your genital hot spots pleasured.

Cheers to that

▶ This position is for all those moments when you just have to get naked and have each other. A high bar stool or loft chair makes for the ideal prop, but the kitchen counter works just as well. Wiggle until your bottom is almost hanging off the edge of the seat, then let your partner support one of your legs so that he can enter you deeply. He will be able to caress your bottom as you hold his body close to yours. The base of his penis will be tight against your clitoris and he will be able to thrust deeply against you. When you get into the groove he can pull your bottom tight up against his pelvis to send you (quite literally) to the edge and beyond.

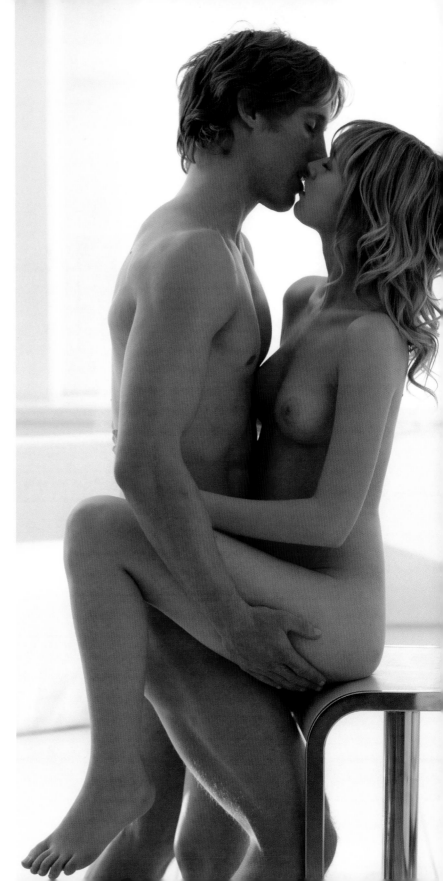

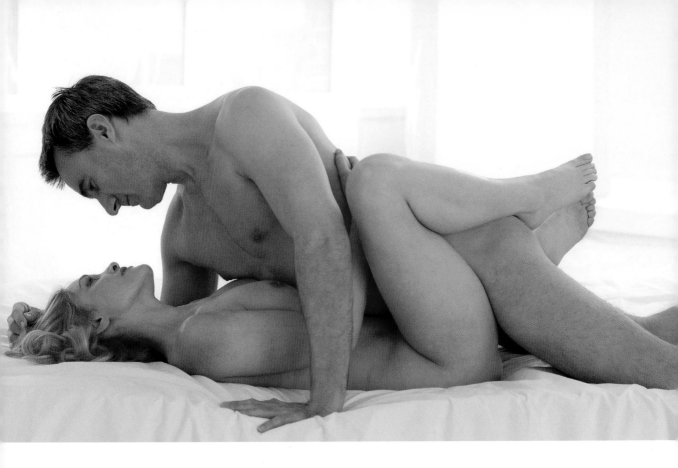

Coital Alignment Technique (CAT)

For women, Coital Alignment Technique is possibly the best thing to ever happen to the missionary position, as it counters that idea that sex automatically means a pistonlike start and lots of activity. CAT takes plenty of patience and practice, and involves a philosophical readjustment and a slower, more relaxed, and perhaps more "feminine" approach to sex. CAT calls for the base of his penis and pelvic bone to stimulate your clitoris so that you receive constant clitoral stimulation. Small, subtle movements are required, together with full-body contact, with focus on the clitoris and pelvic mounds. CAT is good for men, too: rock your pelvis in tune with his and you will build up orgasmic pressure on his frenulum.

Keep a pelvic connection

◀ Lie in the traditional missionary position, but have your partner lift his pelvis up and over your body to enter you. The base of his penis and pelvic bone should tightly fit against your clitoris, and his penis should penetrate you deeply. Maintain constant pelvic contact with a gentle rocking motion, instead of thrusting. To get into a comfortable rhythmic pattern, wrap your legs around him so that you are both moving in perfect harmony.

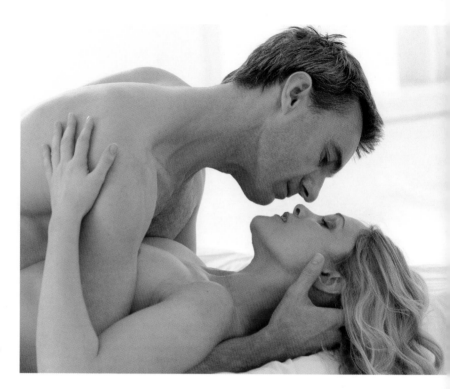

Maintain pressure

▶ Your main goal is for your man to keep up a steady pressure and rub against the area right from your pubic bone down to your vaginal opening. With a little practice, you will soon get into a groove and almost be unable to tell where one of you ends and the other begins.

Enhance the position

▶ You can improve upon this position by squeezing your pelvic floor muscles to increase the friction on your G-spot, and create a tighter vaginal hold on your man's penis. To heighten your, and his, sexual experience and receive a range of sensations, have your partner rock in different directions—first to the left, then to the right, then back to the left again.

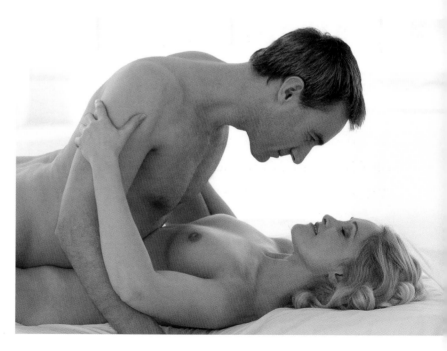

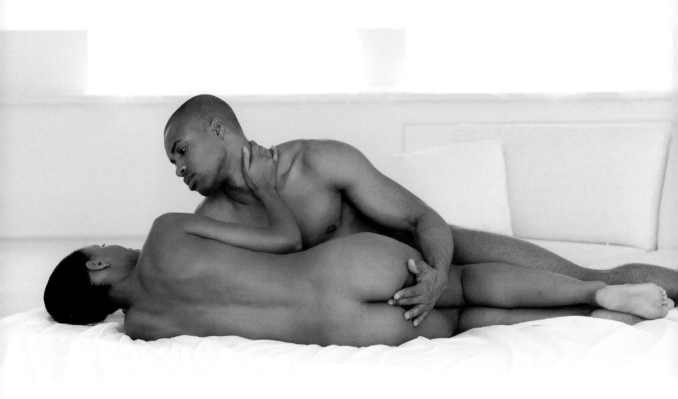

Anal sex

Anal sex can be a healthy and exciting part of a couple's sex life. It is no surprise that most couples have tried out this little-discussed position. Anal sex offers an extension to the usual boundaries of sexual experience; it feels exciting, forbidden, and daring. As a result, it is an instant intimacy enhancer. It also feels really good. This is because the minute nerve endings and perineal sponge in the anus feel great when they are stimulated—so much so that some people even call it "the G-spot of the anus." To enjoy good-quality anal sex, you'll need to feel really aroused and use lots of lubricant. Most importantly: trust your lover, let go of any inhibitions, and allow your body to fully respond to new techniques.

First-timers

◀ If you have never tried anal sex before, start small and low-key. Lie on your side and draw up your legs to make yourself comfortable. Have your partner lie face to face so that he can watch your reactions. It is a good idea if he starts by massaging your labia and clitoris to get you fully aroused and wet. He can then reach over your thighs and massage your perineum and the sensitive area around your anus. Then he can insert a finger or two to get you used to the sensation. You might find that you dislike it, but if you enjoy having your anus penetrated, don't be afraid to keep exploring this new style of sex. Use anal finger-play during conventional intercourse to heighten its excitement for both of you. While penetrating your vagina, your lover can use his fingers to stimulate around and inside your anus. This will give you a very intense orgasm, as all your genital hot spots are brought into play.

Man from behind

▼ One of the best positions for anal sex is a man-from-behind—or spooning—position. To achieve this, ask him to go slowly and set up a signal between you before you start, so you can tell him to slow down or stop. Lubrication is a must because the anus is not self-lubricating. A good way to get started is for your man to perform oral sex. When you are aroused and wet, apply lube generously. At first your man should penetrate your anus with just the head of his penis. He needs to take his time, and you will need to relax and let him in—trusting him is important. He can then move in and out of your anus slowly and smoothly, until he reaches a depth and pace that you find comfortable and exciting. One note of caution: never engage in anal sex followed by vaginal sex since this transfers bacteria, which are likely to cause infection. This holds true for manual or toy play in this region, too.

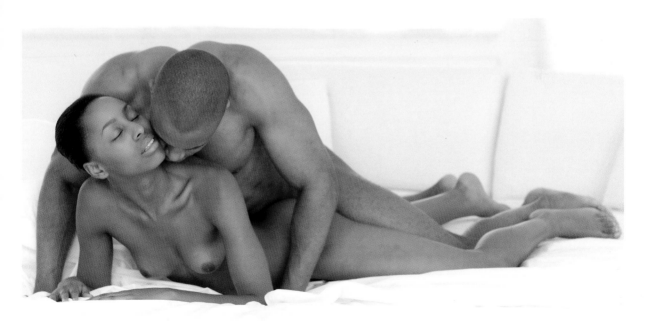

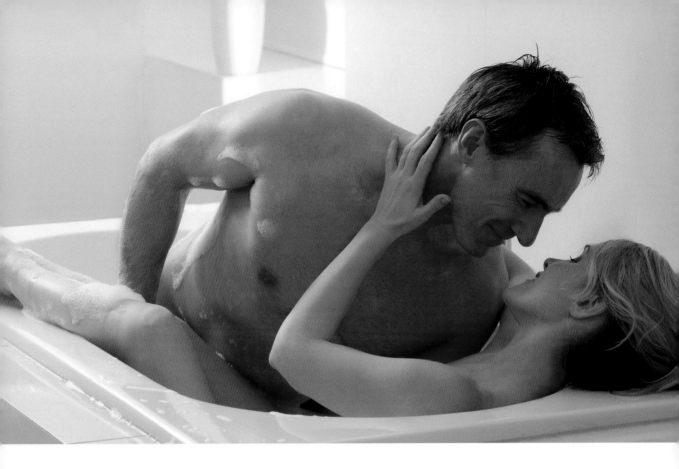

Outside the bedroom

Sometimes all you need to spice up your lovemaking is to vary where you do it. Having sex on a bed is comfortable, warm, and conventional. Sex on your dining room table, in the bathtub, or on the kitchen counter is testing, exciting, and thrilling. You can't just lie back and relax. You have to rethink your position, rhythm, and movement. Having sex outside—or any place where you might get caught—will get your adrenalin running high. You don't have to invite the neighbors over, just add in the possibility of being seen to make your session feel secretly sexy. Make love on the deck under the stars, or entice your man into the bath with you. Be a little daring—after all, sex is meant to take your breath away.

In the tub

◀ Making love in the bathroom gives you plenty of privacy, unlike some other locations around your home, and slipping into a hot bath may be just the relaxing setting you are searching for. Your skin will feel sexily clean. Tubs come in different shapes and sizes, so beware of causing a flood if yours is filled to the brim and you both get in at the same time. Then you can have the discussion about who gets the "faucet end." Of course, if you are lucky enough to own a circular or larger-than-average bath, you may not experience this problem. Run the water nice and warm, and add a little of your favorite pampering bubble bath or foam. Arrange some seductive lighting around the room—tea candles, perhaps—then light some aromatherapy burners for a complete sensory experience.

Standing room only

▶ This is a great position if you and your man like spicing up doing the dishes but aren't in the mood for a workout. Lean against the countertop as your partner stands behind to enter you. This creates the sensation of him holding you. Push your bottom out, then slowly swivel and gyrate your hips against his pelvis as he penetrates. If you are feeling more energetic, you can turn around and plant your bottom on the edge of the kitchen counter. You don't need to remove all your clothes, so it's great for a quickie before your dinner guests arrive. If your sink is in front of a window, don't forget to smile sweetly at your neighbors or passers-by as you reach orgasm.

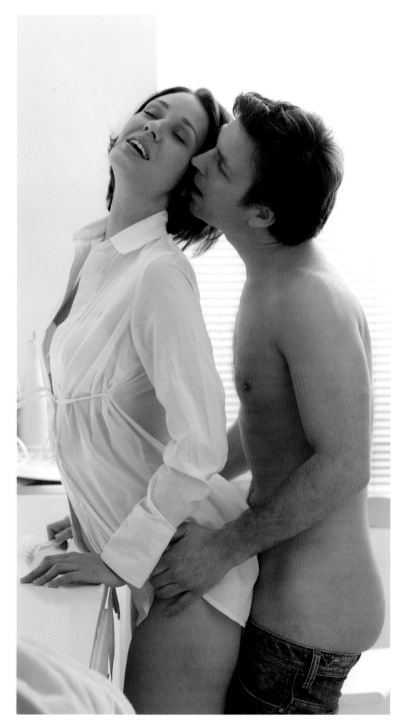

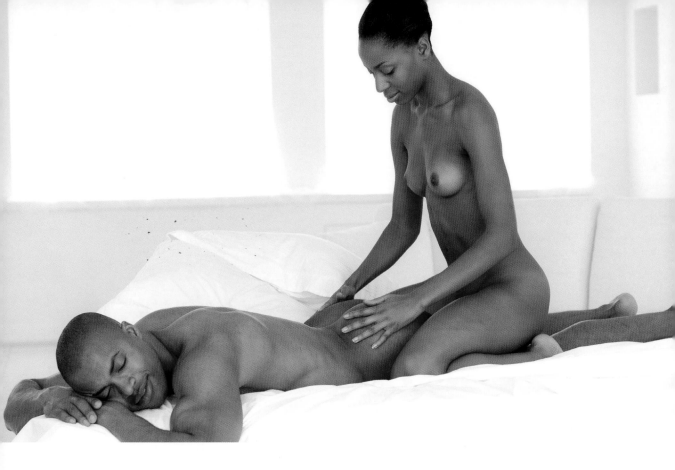

Very erotic, noninsertive sex (VENIS)

There is nothing more intimate than a night of very erotic, noninsertive sex, casually referred to as VENIS. VENIS requires that you get creative with your lovemaking and substitute other erotic activities for penetration. Try naked back rubs, wrestling, bathing or eating food off each other, or sharing fantasies. Include oral and manual sex for added sensual contact. Be a glutton and try everything in one night, or have a weekend of VENIS love. VENIS was created to remind couples that sex should be fun, playful, and intimacy-enhancing. You don't need to have an orgasm, and a session of VENIS will help you and your man luxuriate in each other's touch without feeling too rushed or goal-oriented.

Bare massage

◀ Turn up the heat, strip off, and straddle him. Use a little warmed oil to massage his back and buttocks—he will love being rubbed by you, and the feeling of your naked genitals on the backs of his thighs.

Down for the count

▶ Erotic wrestling is a spicy way to achieve pleasure fast. Most men love to be tested physically, especially when they know that the prize is your body. Challenge him to a little wrestling match and then flirtatiously tell him that the winner takes all. Lube up each other's bodies with massage oil and then slip-and-slide your way to orgasmic bliss. The contact between your oiled-up bodies will create some erotic heat and heighten your sense of touch. You can make it even sexier by telling him that he has to be handcuffed in order to level the playing field—not being able to touch your naked, shimmering body with his hands will amp up his anticipation and heighten his sexual arousal. Just watch out when you take the cuffs off.

A sexual banquet

▶ Whipped cream, honey, and chocolate syrup are all good for licking, kissing, and sucking off each other. Or try feeding him grapes, strawberries, or blueberries—you can use your hands, your mouth, or even your genitals to offer him a feast beyond his wildest dreams. There is also a range of tasty erotic products, including body paint, massage oils, and panties, which are available online.

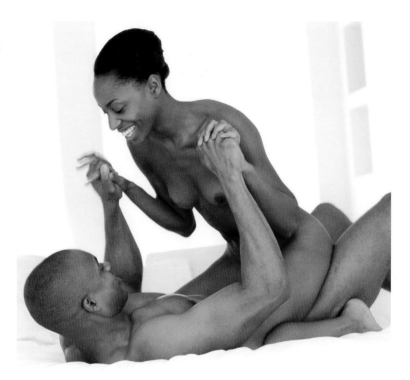

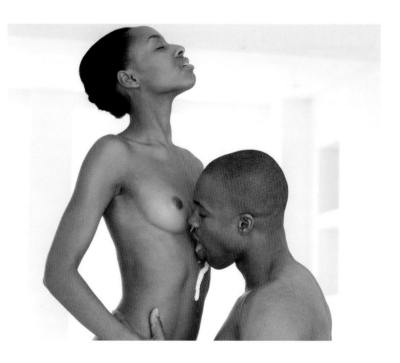

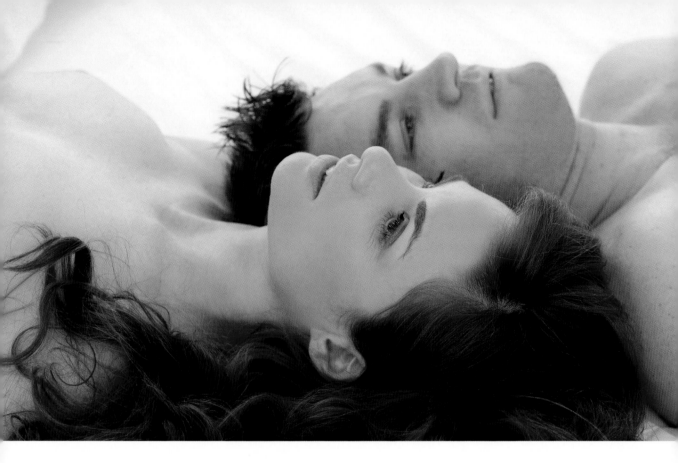

Tantric lovemaking

Tantra is a set of spiritual practices designed to stimulate the senses and make humans more self-aware. Based on the concept that sex is sacred, Tantric lovemaking is about engaging in sex on a deeper level. Breath, touch, and intimate soul-gazing are all key elements. Tantric breath gets you in tune with your body, stroking connects you to each other's sexual energy, and gazing connects you to your lover's spirit. Certain parts of the body—such as the testes and breasts—are believed to be filled with energy and life force, and massaging these areas activates your sexual energy. Use Tantra as a way of reconnecting with your partner after a hectic day or period of separation, and your lovemaking will be energized.

Purifying breath

◀ The breath is a powerful source of energy, and breathing in union can enhance lovemaking. Breathe in through your nose, mouth closed. Inhale slowly so that your stomach rises, followed by your ribs and upper torso. Release the breath completely, mouth slightly parted. Think of your breath as a purifying force, which is cleansing your body with each inhale, and ridding it of toxicity with each exhale.

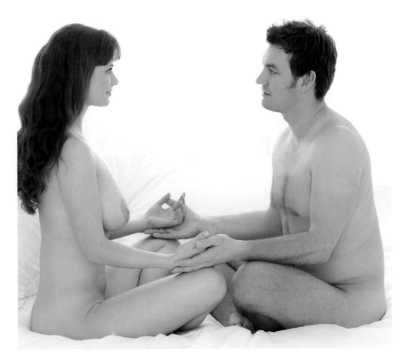

Soul-gazing

▶ This is the practice of looking deep into your partner's eyes and connecting through visual union; this can enhance the quality and closeness of your lovemaking, and all aspects of your life together. Soul-gazing requires you to sit before each other, maintaining eye contact for an extended period—two to three minutes for beginners, but longer as you become experienced. If it feels silly, go ahead and giggle to release tension. You will soon feel more comfortable.

Intimate stroking

▶ Lie side by side, synchronize your breath, and look into each other's eyes. Start stroking each other using gentle, light movements, alternating between a circling action and up-and-down motions. Stroke each other's arms and shoulders, then stroke the neck and back, and finally the thighs and legs, but avoid the breasts and genitals. The goal is to heighten your awareness of each other's bodies beyond the obvious sexual hot spots.

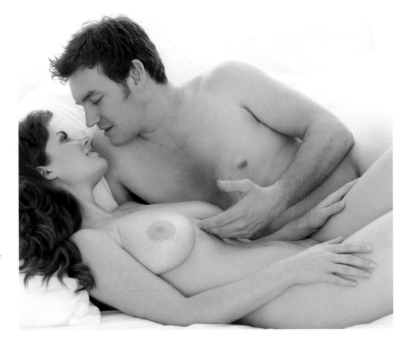

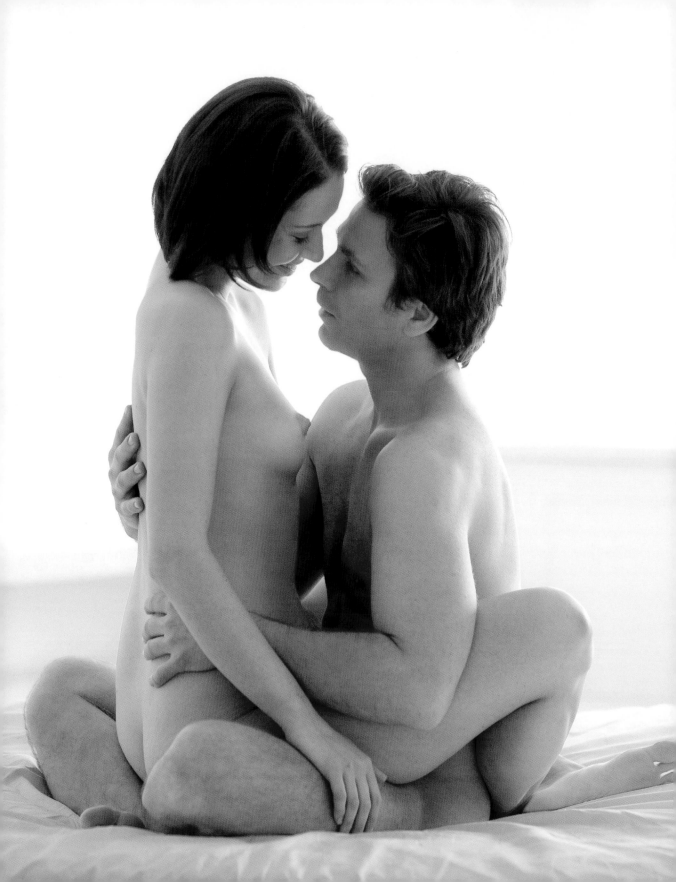

Yab yum

◀ This is the classic lovemaking position in Tantric sex; it allows you both to align your chakras (the wheels of spinning energy running down the center of the body). Sit cross-legged and wrap your legs around your partner. While making love in any position, try implementing a brief period of non-demand intercourse. This is when you stop for 10 seconds while he is inside you. Practice your breathing and let the sexual momentum and excitement heighten to a new level. After this type of delay, orgasms can be especially powerful.

Feel connected

▶ Maintaining eye contact is an important way to feel deeply connected to each other during Tantric sex. By holding each other's gaze, you prevent your mind from wandering, and you make sex a mutual, meditative act.

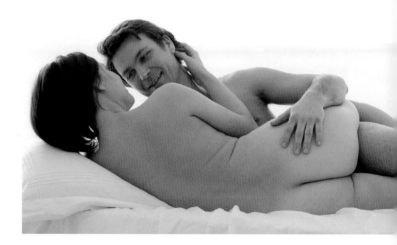

Female energy

▶ Our sexual energy can raise us to a higher level of consciousness, and bring couples closer to the power of a divine source. Many couples find that they enter a heightened state of intimacy with each other and sex becomes imbued with rich emotions and intense sensations. Female energy is revered in Tantric sex and is considered the catalyst for sexual and spiritual transformation. The man honors a woman's sexuality and surrenders himself to its limitless power. Try to escape from your usual roles. If you are used to being submissive during sex, use a woman-on-top position to assert latent dominance and take control of pleasure for both of you.

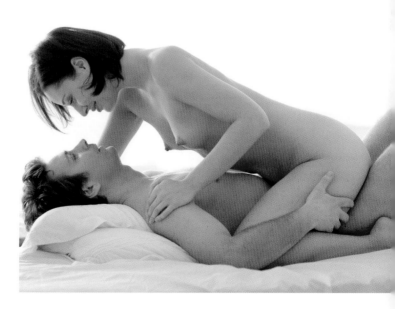

Sex play

Erotica and sex toys are important aspects of sex play. A sex toy is not necessarily only a single girl's best friend. Surveys have found that women in long-term relationships are most likely to use them. This is because sex toys are a fun and erotic way to spice things up in the bedroom. So which sex toy is right for you? From dildos to G-spot stimulators, there is a sex toy for every type of stimulation. There are even undercover-style sex toys shaped like lipsticks or toothbrushes to fit discreetly in your purse.

Age-old toys

Both men and women have had fun with sex toys for millennia, and archeologists have discovered stone dildos (called "olisbos") dating back to 500BCE. In early versions of the *Kama Sutra*, there are references to penis extenders made from wood, leather, and other materials. Even cock rings are not a modern invention—more than 400 years ago, Chinese men used ivory cock rings. As time went by, these were enhanced with extensions to stimulate a woman's clitoris.

Essential accessories

Sex toys are a multibillion, multifaceted business and what was once a secret tool hidden in a woman's dresser is now an essential feminine accessory. If you are uninitiated into the joys of sex toys, now is the time to appreciate the fact that vibrators and other sex toys are actually good for your sex life because they improve your libido and can teach you how to arouse yourself and achieve faster and stronger orgasms.

What's more, you don't have to visit a porn shop to get hold of them, since sex toys now come with online shopping options and discreet packaging. In fact, many women are now turning the traditional Tupperware party on its head by hosting a new, cheeky event: at sex toy parties in each other's houses, groups of friends can admire and giggle over the latest gadgets and erotic novelties, and find their new favorite toy.

Spicing things up

Now that the issue of procuring a sex toy has been settled, you might be worried about how to introduce the idea of using one into your relationship. Don't worry—most men love the idea of spicing things up in the sack. Even so, you should handle this with a little delicacy. Ask your lover how he feels about sex toys, and if he has ever used one with another partner (or even solo). If he seems up for the ride, mention that you would like to try bringing a sex toy into your routine to add a little novelty to your sex life and enhance your relationship.

Reassure him that sex toys cannot replace him, but they can recreate sparks in the bedroom and help you achieve orgasm more easily. Women and men who use sex toys tend to have increased sexual desire and sexual response, and are happier and more satisfied with both their sex lives and lives in general.

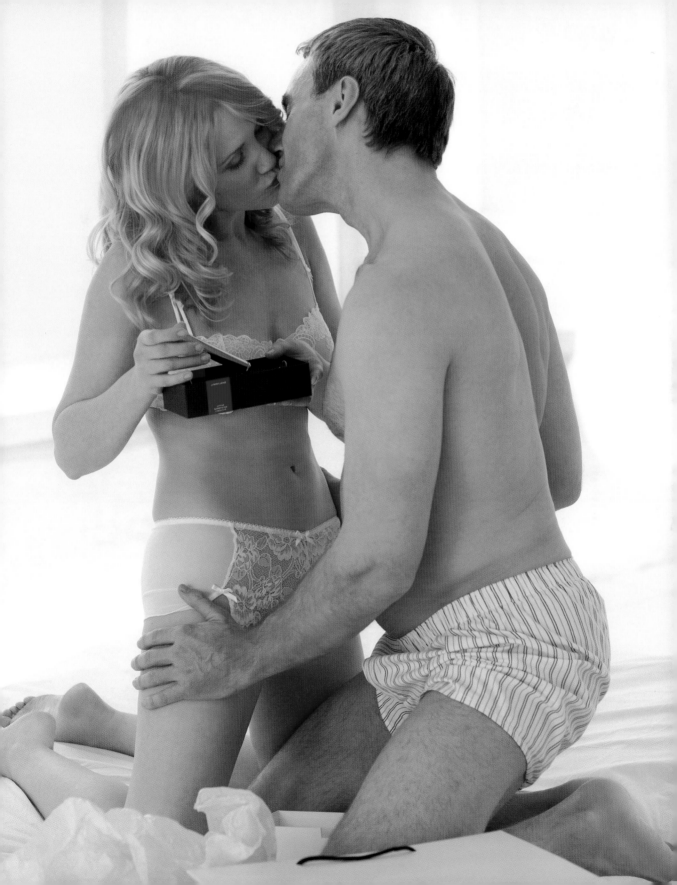

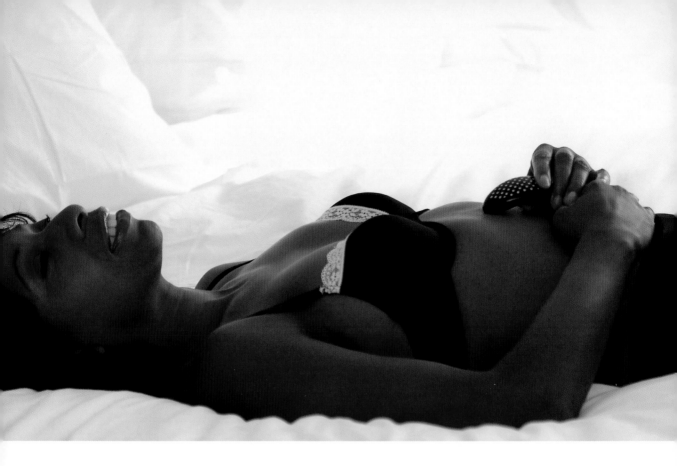

Sex toys

There are toys for all occasions, including vibrators for clitoral stimulation, G-spot stimulators, vaginal exercisers, dildos, and massagers. When purchasing a sex toy, think about what size and type of stimulation you require. Do you want to experience a G-spot or blended orgasm, or have some fun with a pair of vibrating panties? Also ask yourself whether your toy is destined for self play or for use during intercourse—or both. Do a little research before you buy, to find the perfect fit. Thanks to erotica websites, you can purchase all sorts of sex toys without any self-consciousness or embarrassment. You can even choose overnight delivery. Here's every woman's shopping list for sexual pleasure in toyland.

Vibrators

◀ Vibrators are essential toys for
every woman. Look for a vibrator that has
several functions. It should give clitoral
and labial stimulation, or even intra-
vaginally. If you have never used a sex toy
or reached an orgasm during sex, look for
a rechargeable and ergonomically
designed massager. The massaging head
should be flexible so it moves with your
body, and it should come with a couple of
silicone covers to vary the stimulation.
Women who have already mastered
clitoral and G-spot orgasms and want to
experience blended orgasms could try a
G-spot stimulator that also stimulates the
clitoris. G-spot vibrators have a curved
head to help women locate and stimulate
their G-spot. There are also vibrating
penis rings for your lover to wear during
sex for extra stimulation.

Small and discreet

▶ Although there are plenty of lurid and
larger-than-life sex toys on the market,
there are many others, such as the ones
pictured here, that are discreet and easy
to use. Egg-shaped vibrators (top) are
designed for use on the vulva or clitoris,
and can deliver vibrations of varying
intensities, while waterproof vibrators
(second from top) are great for sex play in
the bath. If you like phallic vibrators but
don't want a replica penis, mini-
massagers (third from top) are a stylish
purse-sized option. Or, to hand over
control to your partner, try panties with an
integral vibrator (bottom). Your man
simply operates the vibrator by remote
control—perfect for boring dinner parties.

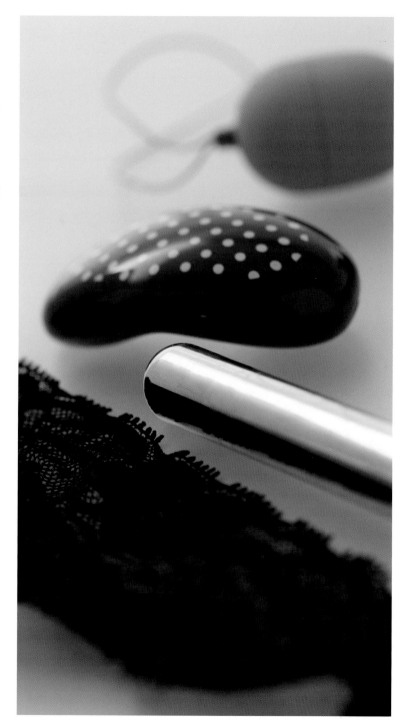

Erotica

Women are starting to embrace erotica. The key is finding which erotica turns you on and gets you in the mood. Whether you are a new couple or in a committed, long-term relationship, erotica can help open your mind to new possibilities in the bedroom. It can expand your awareness of new techniques and positions, and create a dialogue between you about what turns you on. Choose from erotic literature and poetry, magazines, and films—so many options—and use them to fuel your sexuality.

Erotica and self-play

Erotica can also be a good tool for masturbation, with or without a sex toy. Some women struggle to get into a sexy mindset when they have a million things on their mind, but watching an erotic film or reading erotic literature can make those stressors and libido-killers disappear. So the next time you want a fast way to switch off your brain and turn on your body, try using erotica.

Erotic literature

Written erotica is a big turn-on for many women. While men enjoy looking at top-shelf magazines, enjoying the sexy pictures and minimal text, women are more likely to enjoy reading erotica and imagining the visual content themselves. Try reading erotica solo to luxuriate in sexual scenes and the ideas they evoke.

Reading by yourself like this makes the stories feel much more personal. Then, when you want to spice things up with your partner, bring out some of your favorite racy material and read him the X-rated bits. Or get into the habit of reading him an erotic bedtime story—try reading aloud from a collection of real-life women's fantasies. The sound of your voice reading those kinds of words will get his heart pounding, especially if he has free rein to act out the fantasies as you read them aloud. This is a nondemanding, playful way to bring erotica into your relationship without feeling intimidated. It is also a great way to feel relaxed talking about sex to your partner. Reading someone else's words together will help give you inspiration for your own sex talk, as well as providing you with some new ideas for sexual scenarios to act out with your partner.

Reading erotic literature together will inspire your own sex talk, as well as provide you with some new ideas for sexy scenarios to act out.

Erotic films

When most women think of erotic films, we get an image of bleached-blonde porn stars with cosmetically enhanced genitals, raunchy sex scenes, bad dialogue, and nonexistent plots set to cheesy music. Luckily, more women are involved in erotica film production and more and more films are made for women, by women. This means you can count on an engaging plot, sexy men, and even a little bit of romance. The naughty sex parts are still included and will still appeal to men—which means your partner will be just as turned on as you are.

Movie night

Implement a "sexy movie" night, in which you take turns bringing in the erotic movie of your choice. Heat up the popcorn, and snuggle up with your lover in bed or on the sofa for a cozy night in. Make it a fun, intimate experience. Be open to his interests and don't scoff at the films he chooses—he will feel as though you are poking fun at his sexuality and will clam up. Be adventurous and use erotica the way it is meant to be used—to encourage sexy playfulness.

Real expectations

However, it is important to realize that erotica can set up unrealistic expectations for both you and your partner—including what sex should feel like, look like, and sound like. It is rare to find pornography that features real women with normal bodies—and some of the positions and activities are purely for a man's viewing pleasure, not for real life. Looking at this material might also lead to unhealthy body expectations for both of you, so remember to take erotica with a grain of salt. It is sex beautified and glamorized. Men don't usually want to make love to a porn star— the characters and the images erotica projects are merely a starting point from which both of your fantasies can develop.

Reinvigorate your sex life

The images in erotic books and magazines can be a starting point to helping both partners talk about their sexual needs and fantasies. They can also be a valuable source of ideas and fantasies for you both.

If you feel embarrassed or hesitant about bringing erotic material into your relationship, it is worth remembering that it can play a helpful role in enhancing or re-energizing your sex life.

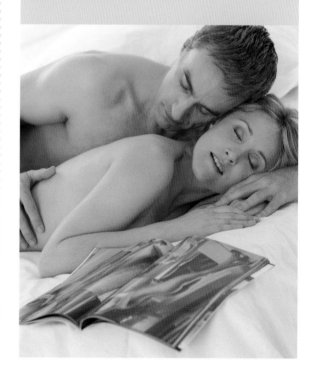

Sex files: Erotic adventures

Erotica and new techniques can add novelty and excitement to a routine sex life, but it's good to discuss them together first. If you're unsure about something, find out about it before dismissing it. This is how one couple addressed boredom and rejuvenated their sex life.

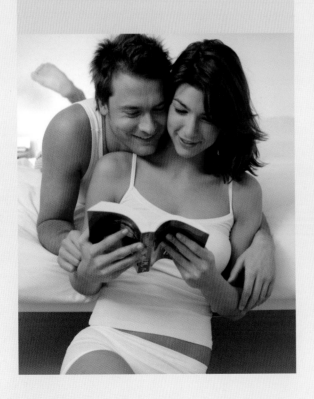

Background

Jan, 27, and Ian, 26, have been together for three years. They are both busy advertising executives. They have a regular sex life and are happy in their relationship.

The problem

Jan and Ian came to see me because Jan was troubled by a sexual request of Ian's. While making love, Ian had asked Jan to put her finger in his anus. Although they are a sexually open couple, Jan felt taken aback, and worried that this signaled a homosexual preference.

Ian had responded by telling Jan that he felt their sex life was getting predictable and he wanted to try something new. "I just want to experiment so we don't get bored. I want to know what it's like to be touched anally during sex." Jan's hesitations remained, but she conceded that they tended to have sex at the same time of day, in the same place, and in the same position.

Finding solutions

An important first step in solving Jan's and Ian's problem was to reassure Jan that anal play is a normal part of a healthy heterosexual relationship. I explained that the anal area is rich in nerve endings and that being stimulated there can feel fantastic. This applies to everyone—male or female, straight or gay.

Once Jan was reassured, we talked about the fact that it's easy to get into a sexual rut and, over time, this can lessen your motivation to have sex. So to reinvigorate their sex life I suggested that Jan and Ian look at erotica together—in the form of books, videos, websites, or magazines. I asked Jan to read some erotic literature by herself. I hoped this would give her the confidence and inspiration to start thinking up her own fantasies. Then she'd be able to bring her own ideas to bed.

As a joint assignment I asked Ian and Jan to get together once a week to share their sexual desires and fantasies. I thought that once they found their sexual "voices" and got used to talking explicitly, they'd find it easy to shake up their sex life.

I also asked them to write down their sexual fantasies on slips of paper and put them in a box. Then, if things started to get dull again, they'd have ideas to draw upon.

What happened?

Jan, who had never looked at erotica before, found it very arousing. After a bit of research, she decided that the idea of anal touching no longer worried her. She also had some ideas of her own to try. She told Ian that she'd often imagined having sex on the desk in his office, and described her fantasy to him in detail, even down to her outfit and the sex position. Ian loved the idea and they decided to enact this sexy scenario at a time when they were sure they wouldn't get caught.

Jan and Ian were excited by their renewed sex life, and as part of their ongoing homework, they made sure that they spent time trying new positions and techniques. As a result, they both felt more able to share their fantasies and desires. They also went online and bought some sex toys, including a vibrator for Jan and a prostate gland stimulator for Ian. "If someone had told me I'd be buying stuff like this a month ago, I wouldn't have believed them," said Jan. "Our sex life has gotten a lot naughtier—and it's great for both of us."

Keeping sex sexy

If you always make love in the same way, or you don't get as turned on as you used to, do something about it. Come up with some sexy ideas that you want to try, and present them playfully to your partner. It could revamp your relationship as well as your sex life.

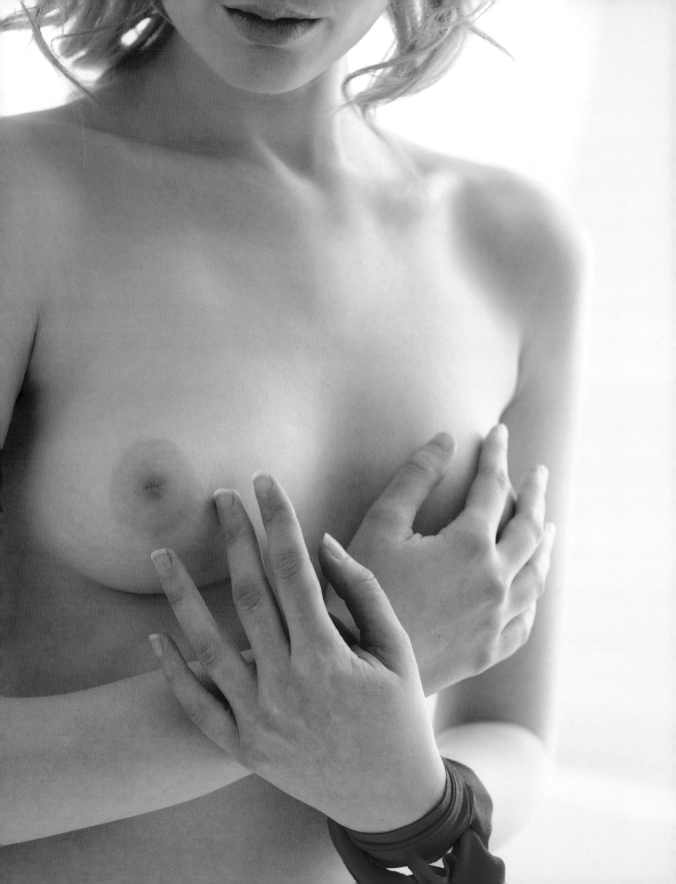

Fantasies

Fantasies nourish your sex life and your relationship. Once you begin thinking about sex and fantasizing regularly, your libido will increase, as will your sexual response. Engaging in role-play is healthy and invites your inner vixen out to play. Fantasies can be as dirty, kinky, and wild as you want them to be. It doesn't mean that you want to act them all out. Some are for your mind; others you would like to become a reality. Let your imagination run riot, and see where it leads you.

Female fantasies

Are you confident in your fantasies, eager to achieve pleasure and revel in the joys of sex? Can you see yourself featuring in your favorite fantasies? By getting in touch with your secret sexual desires, you become more in tune with the woman you want to be, both inside and outside the bedroom. You will also have a lot of fun. Imagination and a few props are all you need for some of the most typical fantasies—escort girl and client, babysitter and parent, doctor and patient—to enter your bedroom.

Healthy fantasy

Despite the benefits of a healthy fantasy life, women sometimes hesitate to engage in fantasy, particularly if it involves someone other than their partner, or sex acts with which they are not comfortable. Just because you fantasize about something or someone doesn't mean that you necessarily want to act it out. For example, women who fantasize about people other than their partners do not want to be unfaithful, they just want to imagine what it would feel like.

This can be helpful to remember if your partner shares a fantasy that you don't necessarily like—just because he fantasizes about having a threesome with you and his favorite female celebrity does not mean he would ever actually consider engaging in it. People often confuse fantasies with unspoken inner needs, but often they are just our mind's way of working out a particular thought or interest. Sexual fantasies shouldn't be taken seriously. Fantasy life is the playground of the mind, so be open-minded, get creative, and start your imagination rolling.

Types of fantasy

When it comes to fantasy, anything goes. Fantasies do not differ so much on a gender level, but on a personality level they definitely do. The one true gender split is that men are more likely to fantasize about being the aggressor, while women are more likely to fantasize about being submissive. Indeed, many women commonly fantasize about being taken against their will. Of course, this doesn't mean that they want to be raped in real life. They may just enjoy the idea of having the control taken from them, or be turned

Let your mind have free rein to go wild. This means no inhibitions, no worries about your fantasies being "abnormal," no holding back.

on by the idea of being so seductive that men cannot resist them. (The idea of not having to put any effort into sex is also appealing!) You wouldn't want to be taken against your will in real life—but to fantasize about it can be fun, safe, and healthy.

Releasing your alter ego

If you never dabbled in theater at school, now is the time to embrace the art of playacting. Think about a character—real or fictional—whom you have always idolized and wanted to emulate. Is it a sexy starlet, a brazen female athlete, a dominatrix, a damsel in distress? Once you dream up your ideal sexy character, give her a name and a personality. What does she look like? What is she like in bed? Is she wild and uninhibited, or ready to learn from her lover? Whatever you dream up, be sure to dress her up—in sexy lingerie or an erotic costume—and then give her free rein to act out her sexual desires in your head. Remember, it isn't you; it's your alter ego, so don't let anything hold you back.

Setting your mind free

This is just as easy: all you have to do is let your mind have free rein to go wild. This means no inhibitions, no worries about your fantasies being "abnormal," and no holding back. However, that can be easier said than done, especially if you have a million other things on your mind.

In order to begin creating a fantasy life, try making time in your schedule to let your imagination quietly meander. Find a comfortable place to relax, then summon up an image of your ideal man. Picture him in detail. Is he tall? Well built? Rough around the edges? A smooth talker? Next, dream up a location—perhaps a deserted island or a cabin in the woods. What happens now is up to you. Once you begin thinking about sex and fantasizing regularly, your libido will increase, as will your sexual response, not to mention the liveliness of your lovemaking.

Dress the part

If you are going to throw yourself into a fantasy role, you will need a sexy costume—the right clothes can transform your personality in seconds. Choose your favorite sexy character and work out what you need to look the part. Search for clothing and props online, in costume shops, or even at your local mall. If you have never worn latex, vinyl, or leather before, here's your chance to reinvent yourself.

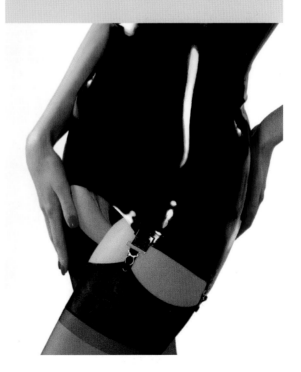

Male fantasies

Male fantasies aren't just about wham-bam-thank-you-ma'am with an attractive women (well, not all the time). Your partner's fantasies are probably as complex as your own. Men fantasize about being in charge, having sex with multiple partners, being tied up . . . some even fantasize about being spanked or spanking their partner. Responding to his fantasies—even if it's just wearing a garter belt or having sex in the closet—will supercharge your sex life and strengthen emotional ties.

Making fantasies come true
When it comes to an active fantasy life, men are the experts. Most men enjoy a healthy enjoyment of pornography and erotica, which makes them pros at conjuring up sexual fantasies. There are a few favorites among male fantasies—such as watching you pleasure yourself—but they are still individual. Perhaps he has a secret fantasy about a certain dress you wear, or perhaps he is dying to see you in a pair of crotchless panties. You'll never know unless you ask.

Indulging his fantasies
How can you make your partner's fantasies come true? If he would like to be dominated, you could buy a pair of handcuffs, a tickling wand, and a blindfold. You could make domination part of your regular sex life or it could be an occasional treat.

Indulge his fantasy about having a threesome by creating your own "third person." Blindfold him and invent the arrival of an imaginary pal. Use running commentary of what you and your imaginary friend are doing to him. Enhance the experience by stroking his body with two distinct types of touch and give him the sensation of a threesome by kissing his lips while using your hands to stimulate him. Using fresh positions or techniques will enhance the newness factor.

Creating a fantasy life
You can help your man create a fantasy life by reading erotica aloud or sharing your own secret fantasies with him while you are both in bed. Try creating a "make your own fantasy" exercise, in which you each supply part of the fantasy. For instance, part of his fantasy might be sex in

Perhaps he has a secret fantasy about a certain dress you wear, or perhaps he is dying to see you in a pair of crotchless panties.

public, and you can add to that fantasy by confessing that you would like to join the Mile High Club by having sex on a plane.

You can also get him going by harking back to his schoolboy days. Who did he fantasize about then—movie stars, his old class teacher? If you help him visualize these fantasies by dressing (and acting) the part, he is likely to be unable to resist and will feel free to let his guard down.

Ready to play?

In order to act out a fantasy, all you need is a healthy sense of adventure and a good sense of humor. It might feel a little awkward role-playing at first, and you may even wonder if you are "doing it right" or if your partner thinks you are acting silly. Don't worry—all men crave a little bit of excitement in the bedroom, so he will love the chance to don a fake name and head off to a deserted isle of adventure with you.

If you already know you want to be a particular character—such as a sexy nurse or an eager-to-please cheerleader—tell your partner about your character in detail. Tell him what she is like, what she wants in the bedroom, and how she is dying to come out and play. No doubt he will respond with his own character—such as a frisky doctor—and the two of you can start to get in the mood. Have a conversation between your characters, in which you "introduce" yourselves and have a little bit of emotional foreplay.

Now is the perfect time for all that creative energy to be put to good use. For instance, why is the nurse alone with the doctor? Is it late at night after everyone has left the hospital? Are you two in a virtually deserted corridor discussing a troubling patient? Does the nurse suddenly drop something and have to bend over erotically to pick it up?

Don't rush into sex. Have fun with your roles and let your imaginations run free. And don't forget: one of his top fantasies is a regular, fun sex life with you, with no crazy bells and whistles.

Embrace the unknown

Many men have fantasies about one-night stands. The notion of having racy, uninhibited sex with a stranger—no strings attached and no real names exchanged—is highly erotic. Why? Because since the sex is anonymous and they know that they will never see the woman again, there are no inhibitions when it comes to trying new things or asking for what they want—sex becomes animalistic and purely pleasure-based.

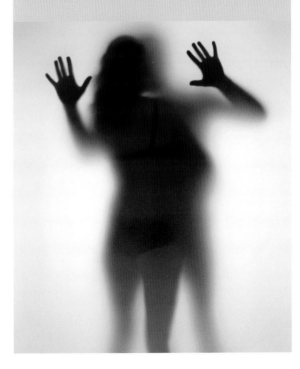

Sharing fantasies

One of the healthiest ways you can add novelty and sexual excitement to your love life is by honestly sharing your fantasies with your partner. Even if you already enjoy a rich and satisfying sex life, you will extend your knowledge and intimacy of each other when you share your best-kept secrets. It might feel disloyal to each other to fantasize about sexual scenarios, but sharing them with your partner will enhance trust and reinforce the strong bond between you.

Safety zone
Sharing your fantasies can be daunting. In order to assuage any worries you have, agree to make your fantasy zone a safe place where you can share your sexual dreams without judgment. Arrangements like this help build the trust and respect you already share in your life together.

Inside the fantasy zone
That said, advise him beforehand that any secret fantasies he might have about your best friend, sister, or mother are best kept under wraps—as are your fantasies about his best friend or brother. Being attracted to attractive people is inevitable, but keep away from fantasies in which feelings might be bruised. It might be tempting to explore his fantasies about the people close to you, but it never ends well.

Avoid mentioning names—he doesn't need to know which movie stars you desire—and just share the events of the fantasy, such as sex in public, on the beach, or on his desk.

Making your fantasies real
Be honest about your feelings. If being spanked, or spanking him, is never going to be an option, say so. If he refuses to don a superhero costume, accept his decision. However, if your partner suggests a fantasy that you would be willing to accommodate, set the rules for fantasy play. For example, maybe you don't want to engage in a threesome, but you would be happy to dress up as a different woman for the night.

Enacting fantasies can enrich many areas of your life. It is both thrilling and erotic to see your imagination take charge in the bedroom.

Build on mutual trust and respect by making your fantasy zone a safe place where you can share your sexual dreams without judgment.

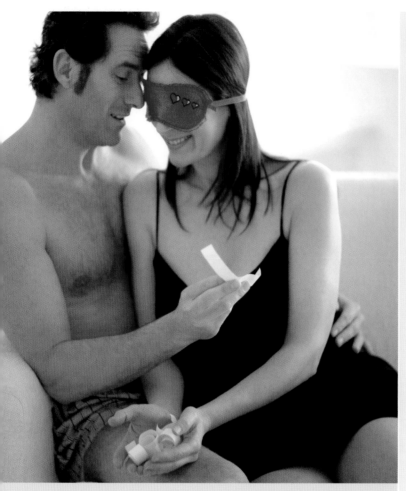

Silver-screen stars

If you want to be on the screen, or your partner enjoys the idea of watching you, he can direct you in a home-style porn movie. Set the scene with romantic lighting and dress the bed with a silk or furry throw. Get into the part with a pair of crotchless panties and high heels, then start acting. Caress your body, moan loudly, and use a sex toy or vibrator to pleasure yourself. After you have finished filming, watch the tape together and let the arousal start all over again.

Strangers in the night

Recreate the butterflies from the first time you met your lover by meeting all over again. Meet him at a bar or hotel wearing a new outfit, new make-up style, and even a wig. Be creative and keep it sexy by picking a fake career, fake name, and fake life story. It is a great opportunity to be that blonde flight attendant who is dying to lose her virginity, or that sexy redhead career woman who can't wait to dominate a man in bed.

Teacher's pet

If you still fantasize about being seduced by one of your old college professors, recreate the scene with your partner. Dress in a pretty dress and kitten heels for your tutorial with him. He invites you into his office and tells you that he is impressed with your latest piece of work. You smile a bit and accidentally show him some thigh. He offers you a drink and sets out to seduce you. It's your first time, so you're a bit nervous, and you'll both have to be very quiet because there are classes being taught next door.

Fantasy box

Share your fantasies by writing them onto slips of paper and putting them in a fantasy box. Select a slip of paper and have fun acting it out. Experiment, too, with the ideas given here: "silver-screen stars" inspire home-movie-style fantasies, while "strangers in the night" and "teacher's pet" bring to life common fantasies you may already entertain.

Sex files: Sexual role-playing

Fantasy and role-play can be an effective method for couples to "switch off" from the grind of daily life and feel sexy again. By playing different roles you can actually get in touch with your own real sexuality. This is how one couple used fantasy to jump-start their floundering sex life.

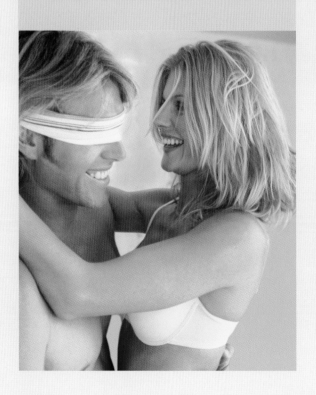

Background

Meredith, 32 years old, is a financial attorney. Her job is very demanding and she spends almost 80 hours a week at work. Kyle, 34 years old, is a salesman who does much of his work from the road or from his home office. They've been together for eight years and, despite their ups and downs, want to stay together. Kyle works fewer hours than Meredith and has a more casual lifestyle and relaxed attitude towards work.

The problem

Meredith said she couldn't remember the last time when she "properly" enjoyed sex or felt truly sexy. She said she always found it difficult to switch off from work. "When Kyle and I have sex, it tends to be late at night—I usually try to have an orgasm quickly just so I can go to sleep and feel OK in the morning."

Kyle said that he was starting to find Meredith's brisk and mechanical approach a turn off. "Sometimes it's like she just can't loosen up, even after a glass of wine. Sex feels robotic—I penetrate her, she has an orgasm, and then I ejaculate. It all functions OK, but I can't say it's sexy."

When I asked Meredith and Kyle if they had a healthy fantasy life, they both scoffed. "A fantasy to me would be a day off work to do whatever I wanted," said Meredith, "Or better yet, a whole week off," Kyle said.

Finding solutions

After explaining to Meredith that it is normal to struggle to switch off during sex, I suggested that they both try fantasizing while making love. This would stop Meredith from thinking about her to-do list or court dates. And it would help Kyle stop monitoring Meredith's mechanical sexual style. When Meredith asked what fantasy she should think about, I asked her to come up with an idea of her own.

After some hesitation she said she liked the idea of being "taken" by Kyle. "I'd like him to be in total control of my body with no work on my part. It would be amazing to be completely submissive."

Kyle loved the idea—he said that he'd had fantasies of being dominant before, but hesitated to reveal them for fear that he would seem sexually aggressive.

I explained to Kyle and Meredith that S&D (submission and domination) is a common fantasy that many couples love to act out in bed. It doesn't have to signal a desire for aggression or subservience in any other area of life. To get them into their respective dominant and submissive roles, I suggested that they use handcuffs and a blindfold. I also advised them to create characters for themselves—this is usually a fast way to release inhibitions. Meredith, for example, could be a submissive employee, and Kyle could be her disciplinarian boss.

What happened?

At our final session, I asked Kyle and Meredith to tell me about their role-play experience. Meredith said, "It felt good to surrender and to be totally in Kyle's hands. It made me realize how controlled I am most of the time." Kyle, meanwhile, loved feeling like he was in control of their sex life. He enjoyed being able to tap into the dominant side of his personality, which he doesn't often get to express around Meredith. The couple were so excited about role-playing that they decided to devote one night a month to pure fantasy. "As well as the eroticism, it's a big relief to escape from our day-to-day personalities," said Meredith.

Express your wild side

Fantasies are a way of giving your sexuality free range to break out of your—and his—usual modes of behavior. Just be sure to set boundaries of open-mindedness and respect, then you and your partner can have a rich, playful fantasy life that fulfills both of your needs.

Dressing up

Dressing the part and role-playing are opportunities to let your fantasy life manifest itself. You and your partner have the opportunity to wear clothes and use accessories—a feather boa, a fireman's helmet, a stethoscope, or thigh-high boots—that are not part of your day-to-day life. Playing at being another character gives you and your partner a break from your traditional roles—husband, wife, parent, employee, or boss. Start with characters that suit your personality, and then become more adventurous.

Revel in role-play

Role-play has many benefits for your love life—it extends your sexual boundaries and keeps your relationship exciting. Role-play is good for all types of romantic relationships, but if you have been with the same partner for a number of years, creating your favorite fantasy gives you both a safe way to make love to another character without hurt feelings or negative consequences.

Sometimes all you need is a few props to kick-start your fantasy life. A bustier makes you feel like a call girl, motorcycle boots turn you into a biker babe, and a fireman's hat turns your man into a local hero. Keep an open mind and an eye out for provocative props. They don't have to be expensive; in fact, the simpler the props, the better—think feather duster and naughty maid, or bunch of grapes and slave girl or boy.

Lingerie with character

Purchase some bedroom-only lingerie—sexy underwear and accessories that lend you a character. A vampy leopard-print bodice and a pair of heels give you a sense of being uninhibited. Frilly, romantic underwear makes you feel virginal. Pasties and a G-string bring out the stripper in you, and leather and latex create the dominatrix. Add a little spice to everyday life by keeping your undergarments sexy—it can be a secret shared by you and your partner. You will feel sexy and it might turn you into a seductress after a hard day in the office.

Chaps and cowboy hats

The next stage is dressing up and costume. For instance, if you are into NASCAR, dress up in a racing-girl uniform. Leave the jumpsuit zipper

Kick-start your fantasy life with a few props. A bustier makes you feel like a call girl, motorcycle boots turn you into a biker babe.

undone to reveal a girly lace bra or glittery tattoo. If cowboys and westerns make you wild, buy a hat and chaps and leave them lying around for your man to find, then enter the bedroom wearing a saucy cowgirl-style costume.

With costumes picked out, choose character names for yourselves and create an appropriate context in which the action is set. For example, are you a glamorous starlet who is dying to get it on with her sexy co-star onscreen? Are you an innocent snow bunny who got lost on the trails and needs a hot ski instructor to guide you back to your room—where he will draw you a bath, and help you get out of your cold, wet clothes?

They might sound silly at first, but only you and your partner will hear these stories, so be as adventurous and free-spirited as you feel inclined. Fantasy is freedom: give your character a sexy name, a wig, and dramatic fake eyelashes. When you have become adept at acting out your preferred fantasy types, keep on being inventive with the characters and extending the role-play.

Sexy scenarios

Once you and your partner are comfortable with the characters and scenes you want to explore, you will probably find it helpful to create a scenario to enact—ideas of how the story between your fantasy alter egos unfolds.

For example, maybe you want to play escort girl and client. Arrive at the front door or the bedroom decked out in a cheap miniskirt, high-heeled stilettos, red lipstick, and fishnets. You will have spent some time creating your character, so when your partner answers the door, you will be ready to introduce yourself in character, and state your terms of payment in a convincing manner.

Your partner needs to go along with the performance, but he will probably respond to your flirtatious glances by being unable to keep his hands off you. Try to stay in character throughout the scenario, even if you want to giggle.

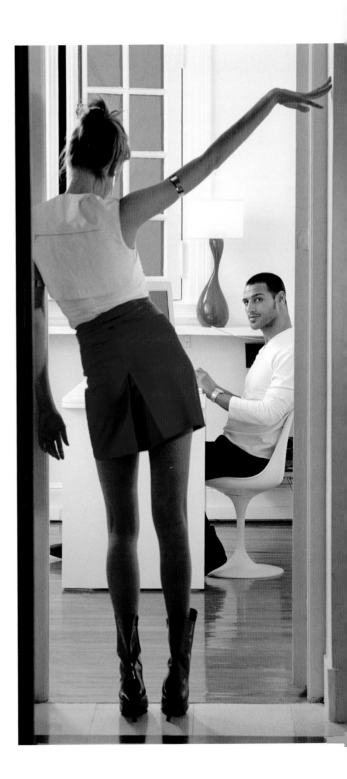

Strip show

Men love strip clubs—no doubt about it. And why wouldn't they love watching sexy, scantily clad women grinding on stage for their viewing enjoyment? For a special treat, recreate this sexually charged environment in the comfort of your own home. Simply pick a time when you will have the house to yourself, light the room appropriately, dress the bed with a velvet throw, play some music you can dance to, and invite your man in to view his very own personal strip show.

Fool-proof stripping

How can you act the part of a sexy dancer and still feel confident? Realize that virtually whatever you do that involves stripping will turn your man on—which means that reinventing yourself as a burlesque star is a lot simpler than you think.

Star turn

Confidence is sexy. This might explain why the thought of a half-naked woman dancing for other people's viewing pleasure is so erotic—it takes confidence to put your body and sexuality on display in such an uninhibited way. If you want to get into the role, you might find it helpful to dress the part by wearing nipple tassles or even crotchless panties. If your partner is accustomed to you taking a less-than-confident sexual role, he will be impressed to see you take center stage.

Dancers are known for their dramatic make-up, so glam up your look by wearing thick fake eyelashes, glittery eye shadow, and daring red lipstick. You can also use make-up to fake a dancer's body—bronzer between your breasts creates the illusion of deep cleavage, and light shimmery body powder down the middle of your shins makes your legs appear thinner and longer.

Set the scene

Dim the lights or arrange candles right around the room to subtly light your body. This can help make you feel more confident—since you won't be standing under the glare of electric lighting—and create the dusky atmosphere of a strip club.

Choose the music wisely. The best music for dancing and stripping is the kind that makes you feel happy and confident. Whether this is a

Reinventing yourself as a burlesque star is simpler than you think—virtually anything you do that involves stripping will turn your man on.

classic hit or a romantic slow number, find one that fits you, rather than trying to fit yourself to the music. Just make sure it has a good beat and is not too fast for you to dance to.

Get into the role

To get the moves of a striptease dancer, just remember what your mother taught you—about posture, at least. Keep your back straight, hold your head high, and smile—not only will this help you relax and exude confidence, it will also keep your tummy tucked in and your breasts out. Pointing your toes will elongate your legs and make cellulite disappear. Wear stilettos to show off your legs and your toe cleavage.

Private dancer

Maintain eye contact with your lover throughout and keep your hips moving seductively. Smile softly and shyly bite your lip as you unhook your bra. Once you have removed it, return to dancing in front of him and then move on to the next piece of clothing. When he can contain himself no longer, strip off your panties. Remind your man that most strip clubs don't allow fraternization between clients and dancers, but tell him that you are ready to break the rules for him. Slowly grind your body against his crotch.

When he can't take the anticipation any longer, tell him the only tip that you require is sex with him. He'll get his pleasure, but you will also get to call the shots and have sex exactly the way you like it. Take this opportunity to show him some of the moves you enjoy.

Paid pleasures

Turn the tables and play with the idea of paying your man for private pleasures. Indulge in a little male-escort or sexual-slave fantasy. You could demand oral sex, an erotic massage, or some S&M—handcuff him to the bed—or even get him to perform a strip show of his own.

Enjoy yourself

Strip one piece of clothing off at a time and enjoy yourself. Take your time and show your man different views of your body—your back, your legs, and your bottom—by turning around as you dance. When you get down to just your bra and panties, walk over and give him his very own lap dance. As you move your body, caress your skin seductively. Enjoy showing him how sexy you are. Let him look, but not touch.

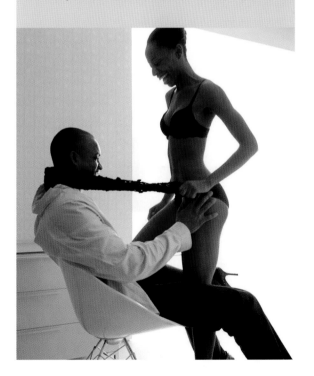

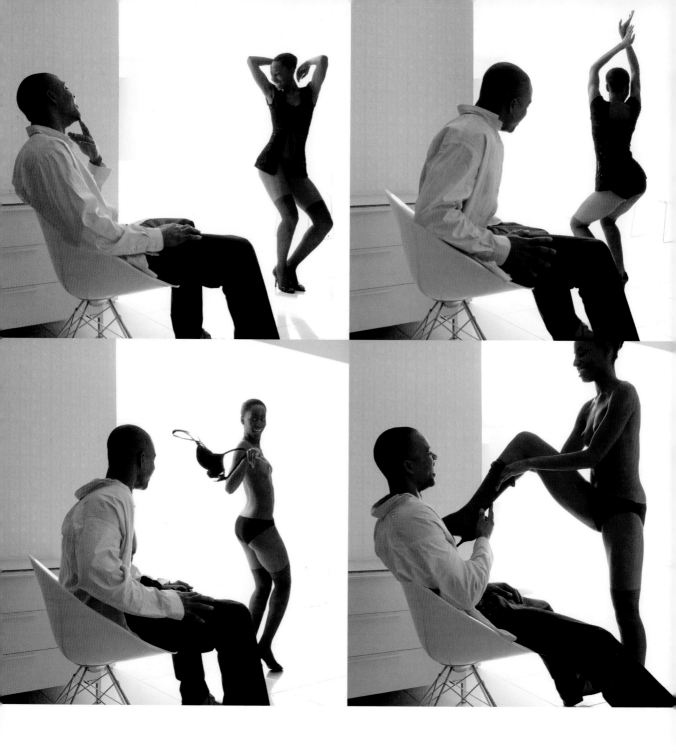

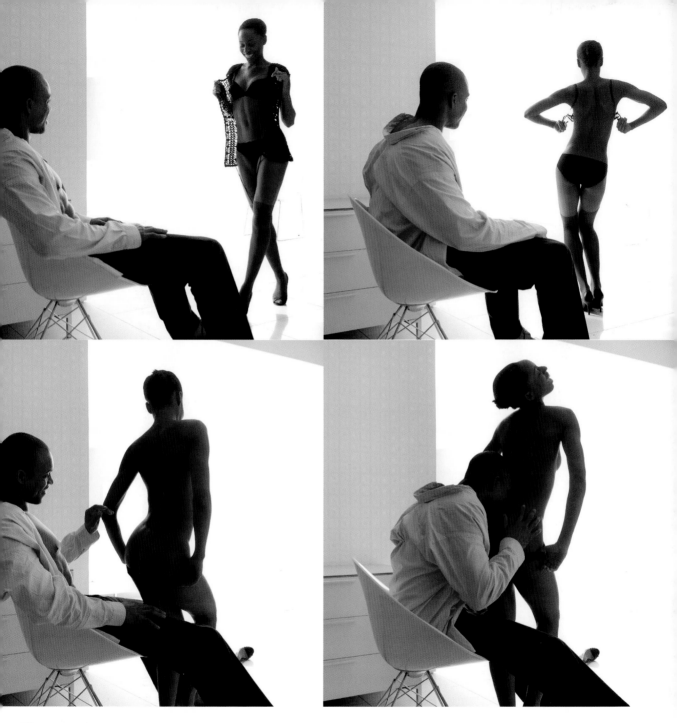

Your striptease routine

▲ Set up the scene to suit yourself, and pay special attention to lighting and atmosphere. Make sure that you are the one that calls the shots throughout. Be in control—he'll love it. Play music that turns you on, and that you enjoy and can dance raunchily to. It will be sure to turn him on, too. Above all, keep your sense of humor intact!

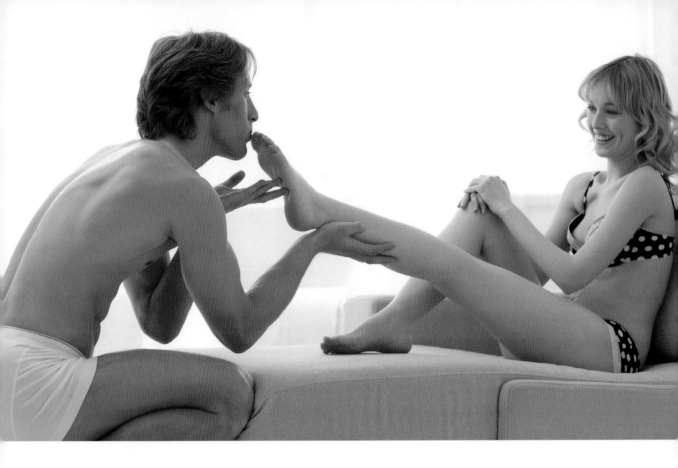

Submission and domination

When submission and domination are mentioned, most people visualize sado-masochism (S&M). However, S&D is not so extreme and is much less intimidating for couples wanting to dabble in power games. S&D is a wild, sexy-romp departure from traditional routine, and brings sex back to its most animalistic, instinctual form. It can still be light-hearted, fun, and even romantic, but S&D takes away the pressure of "lovemaking" because it is more about need-fulfillment. Most people enjoy a little bit of both worlds, so take turns giving and receiving pleasure or pain. There are lots of sexy scenarios—butler and mistress, au pair and parent, master and courtesan—so let your imagination go wild.

Queen for a night

◀ Play the dominating diva for the night and have your love-slave do your sexual bidding. Choose a name that you would prefer to be called—such as "Queen"—and demand to be obeyed. Insist that he strip to his underpants, but reward him with a smile if you enjoy his sexy foot massage. Switch between being adoring and strict, if you want to keep him alert and obedient to your whims.

Tantalize him

▶ S&D doesn't have to involve pain, but you can choose to administer or receive punishment as part of your role. This might include tickling him with a feather, spanking, or using handcuffs or hot wax. Agree beforehand on acceptable treats and punishments.

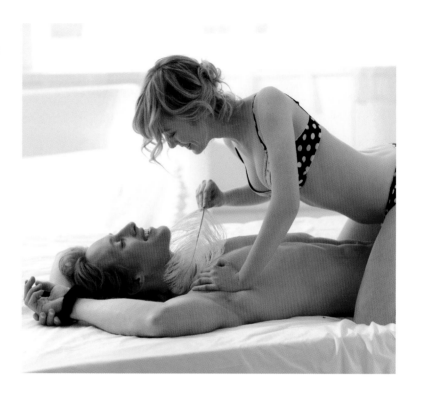

Submit to him

▶ Acting the sexual submissive can be fun, too. The prospect of not having to take the initiative can be quite appealing to most people. Sexual submissives can act out their role painlessly through giving massage, watering the garden, cleaning the house in a maid's uniform, or cooking dinner in the nude. If you are a good girl, your lover might reward you with oral sex—although a blindfold will remind you that he is still in charge. For misbehaving, he might "punish" you by insisting that you have sex with him, or by demanding fellatio or another sexual treat. You can get your own back when it is your turn—insist that your slave scrub the bathtub, and spank him if he gets impudent.

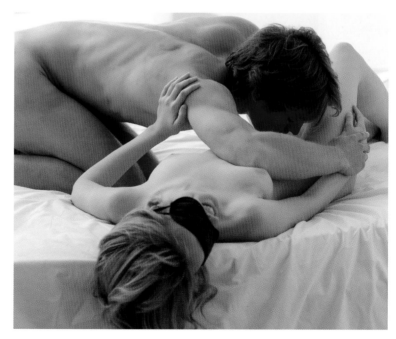

On location

Since most fantasies take place only in the mind of the fantasizer, the location tends to be as wild as the fantasy itself. From a beach in Belize to a balcony overlooking the Rhine, from a raft lost at sea to a Hollywood movie set, fantasy locations are not always easy to access in real life. However, there are many fun and sexy ways to recreate fantasy locations in your bedroom, and beyond. With a few props and some imagination, the scene of any fantasy location can be brought to life.

Trains, planes, and automobiles

Okay, you are not supposed to have sex in any of these places—unless you have booked yourself a couchette on the overnight sleeper—but it shouldn't stop you from enjoying sex on the run. Pretend to be strangers who have just met, or secret agents on a mission, then take your aroused selves off home or to a handy hotel room to finish what you started.

Alternatively, if you have a long road trip ahead of you, plan a few diversionary stops. Park in a deserted spot and have sex in the back seat. Indulge in a hitchhiker fantasy, imagine he's a racing driver and you are a groupie, or pretend to be a teenager borrowing Dad's car for the night.

Outdoor sex

If you want to act out a fantasy of having sex in public, get yourself into the exhibitionist state of mind with some public displays of affection. You don't have to go all the way—just a make-out session in public might give you the adrenalin rush you crave. Then take your passion back to the safety of your own home, and add to the thrill of daring sex by doing it with the lights on or in the confined space of a closet or under-stairs

cupboard. Pretend that you have to rush in case you get caught, or add to the intensity of the experience by pretending that you aren't allowed to make any noise in case someone hears you.

Alternatively, go for a run in the park with your partner. When you've got your heart pumping and worked up a sweat, pull your man into a clump of bushes for some hot and heady lip-locking.

Fantasy island

Another idea is to recreate the famous fantasy of sex on the beach. Barring sex in the playground sandbox, you can bring some island romance into your bedroom with Brazilian samba music, the scent of suntan lotion massaged into your and your partner's skin, and sexy swimwear for you both. Island-themed drinks with umbrellas are a nice touch. If you have any pictures or video of you at the beach, use these as background reminders to get you in the mood.

Pretend you are a sexy tourist who is looking for an island romance, and your partner is the islander who is always ready to show a pretty holiday-maker around town. Or you could swap roles and let him be the visitor while you act the part of the pretty island girl in a coconut bra.

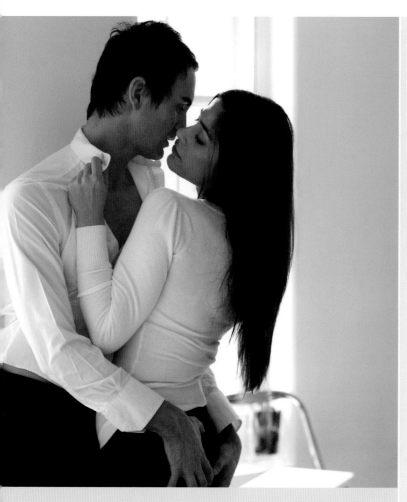

Prime locations

Once sex is liberated from the bedroom, you will find that almost any location—from the most seemingly banal of places, such as the much-trodden staircase in your home, to the plushest of luxury hotel rooms—could be great for spicing up your sex life. Try these ideas, to start—and you might just find that the world, as they say, is your oyster.

Stairway to heaven

Believe it or not, the steamiest fantasy location could be the stairs. The next time your partner tries to slink off to bed early, ambush him on the stairs, rip his clothes off, and take him there and then. Whatever position you assume, the stairs will give his penetration a whole new angle. Add a little frisson of excitement: don't use your home staircase—borrow someone else's.

Under canvas

Camping is not most people's idea of a dream date, but making out by the light of a campfire is definitely the stuff of fantasy locations. Prepare the scene with blankets—and, yes, insect repellent—then enjoy sex under canvas. You will have to be quiet because tents aren't very private—or make as much noise as you want and annoy the neighbors. Use the opportunity to role-play—think caveman meets cave girl, or intrepid explorers lost and alone.

Luxury places

Who isn't turned on by the idea of sex in a luxurious hotel room or on board a yacht or ocean liner? If it is within your budget, book yourselves into a five-star room for the night. Enjoy the smooth sensation of expensive sheets against your skin. If the room has a balcony, have sex on it while you enjoy the view. If pricey hotels are not an option, create similar luxury at home with soft lighting, candles, and a bottle of bubbly. Switch off the phone, send the children to stay with their grandparents and enjoy the luxury of one-on-one time with your lover.

Fetishes

Fetishism is a sexual attraction to objects or actions. The term comes from the word "charm," and was originally used to refer to talismans and good-luck items. This definition still holds true—except that a sexual fetish is one in which a person believes that an object or material is infused with sexual attraction rather than good luck. Many people find that fetishes add spice and excitement to their sex lives. Some common examples include underwear, shoes, and items made of rubber or leather.

Personal attractions

Fetishism might bring to mind social deviance, but most of us have fetishes we are not aware of. A man may describe himself as a "breast man" or "bottom man." Other people find that they are attracted to certain hair colors or lengths. Many objects have been infused with incredible sexual power by the media—the little black dress, stilettos, the tuxedo, red lipstick, chocolate, luxury cars, motorcycles, leather jackets, and champagne, for instance. These items are glamorized and sexualized, and are accepted as part of most of our fantasy lives.

Common fetishes

Many people are attracted to and aroused by different types of slippery and smooth materials, such as vinyl, leather, silk, or latex. The sensation of skin against satin or silk sheets is very erotic. Fetishes for vinyl or latex are suggestive of sexual deviance and are a popular part of S&M play.

Common S&D fetishes might involve spanking, restraints, punishment, and lack of control or taking charge of someone. Bondage fetishists have an attraction to gags, handcuffs, and chains. This might also include leashes, collars, and masks and generally involves S&M play.

Talking dirty to your partner during sex is also a common fetish behavior. This might range from a few moaned words to verbal abuse—either giving it or wanting to receive it—in order to get excited or reach a climax.

An exhibitionist fetish involves sexual satisfaction from being watched during sex or masturbation. This might include having sex in public places or in other locations where there is

The media have fetishized many objects: the little black dress, stilettos, the tuxedo, red lipstick, chocolate, luxury cars, leather, and champagne.

a risk of being seen. Alternately, a voyeuristic fetish involves sexual enjoyment from watching others, either in person or via pornography.

A more unusual fetish involves bodily fluids such as urine. The fetishist, usually drawn to the earthiness of the smell, taste, or texture of these substances, might get pleasure from drinking the fluids or rubbing them on the skin.

Discover yours and his

Many women and men have a fetish for shoes—think sexy high-heeled boots or stilettos. Women love collecting, wearing, and categorizing them. Men love watching women wearing them. If he has a thing for high heels, your man will find it very arousing when you wear them in the bedroom. Show off your long legs, let him smell and caress the leather, and taunt him with your toe cleavage.

Many men are aroused by the idea of glossy red lipstick being smudged across a woman's face during sex, most likely because they associate it with pornography and wild, uninhibited sex. Tie him to the bed with a silk scarf and tease him with your red lips. Leave lipstick smudges on his chest and face.

Be more daring, and play with exhibitionism and voyeurism. Tell your partner you want him to secretly watch you while you masturbate in the shower. Enjoy the sensation of being the object of his secret desire.

Fetish play

There are hundreds of different fetishes and they vary from person to person. Fetishes can be a healthy and acceptable way to enhance sex, as long as you both enjoy what you are doing. However, when the fetish itself becomes the primary sexual focus or a requirement for sex, then it creates an unhealthy balance in your sex life. This caveat aside, don't be afraid to explore new things—but keep it fun.

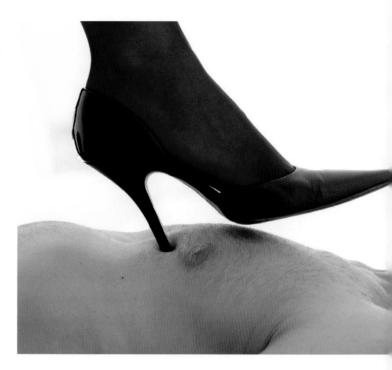

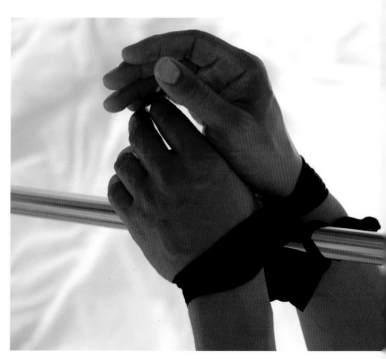

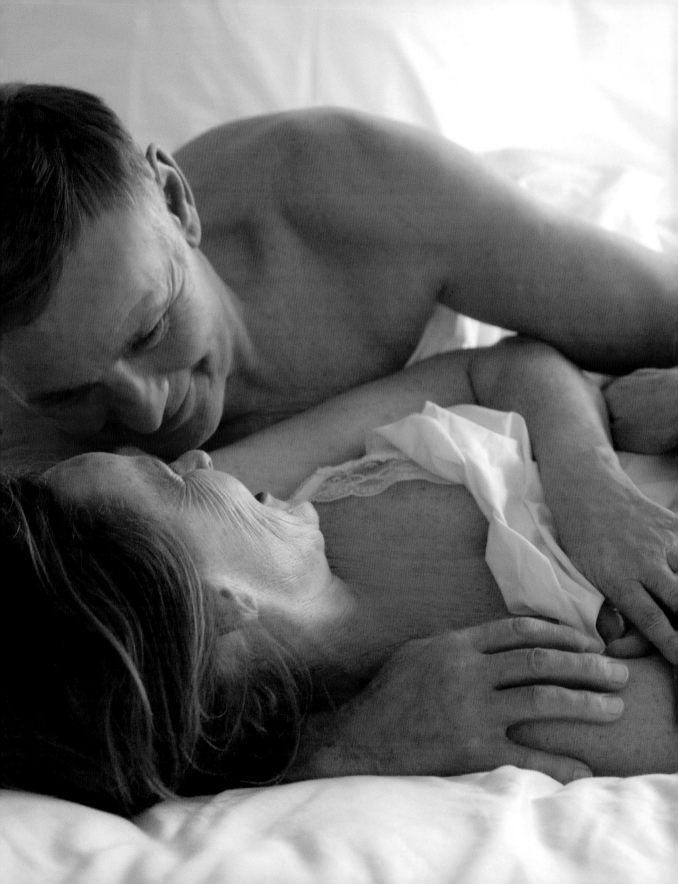

healthy sex

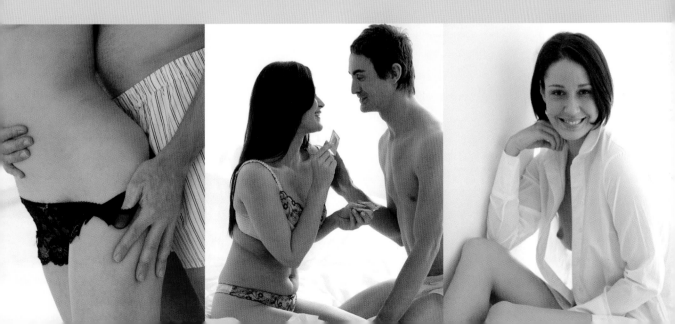

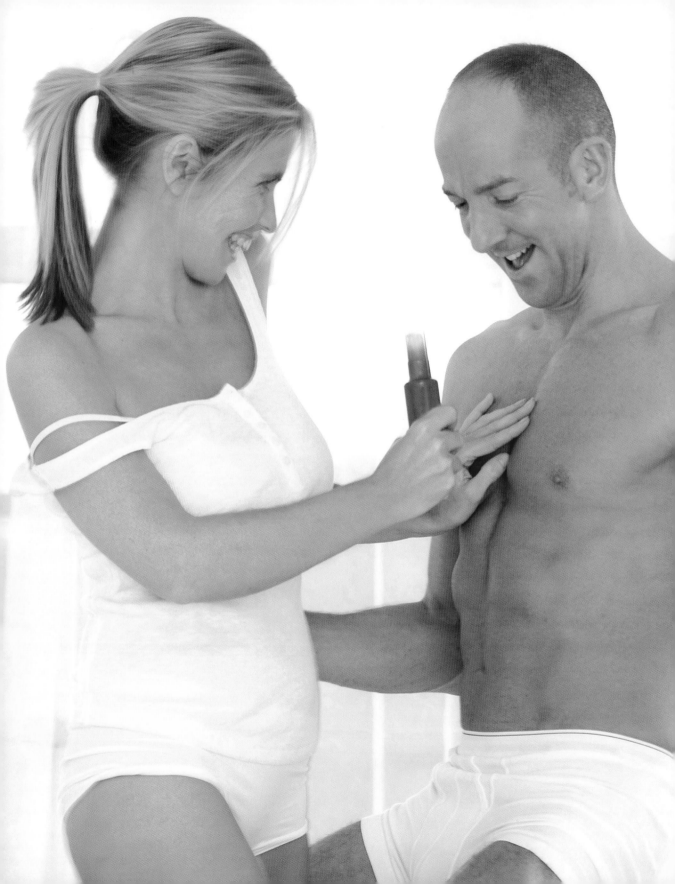

Sexual health

Real sexual health requires women to be unafraid to seek great sex. Emotional distress, sexual difficulties, or dysfunction can be hard to discuss, even with a compassionate doctor, so you need to be bold and brave. Don't be afraid to ask questions, request a second opinion, or learn about your inner workings—physical and mental. Sexual health is all-encompassing and looking after it means taking care of your body, your mind, and your relationship. The path to improved sexual health takes time and attention, but the reward is increased happiness, so it is always worth it.

A healthy body

A great sex life requires a healthy body and that means more than just exercising regularly and eating a nutritious diet. A healthy body is the result of a fit mind, a fit lifestyle, and a commitment to sexual health. Whatever your age or stage of life, a healthy body will help you achieve a satisfying sex life. Our bodies shape our sexual experience and enjoyment, so taking care of our health should be one of our top priorities. Care for your body, and watch your sex drive soar.

Healthy weight

What does a healthy body look like? The view most commonly presented by the media is that a healthy body is a very thin body. However, if you ask your doctor, he or she will tell you that a healthy body is one that has a safe body mass index (BMI)—typically between 18–24—and a waist measurement of less than 35 inches for women and 40 inches for men. Most internet health sites include a BMI calculator. (A healthy weight range is always unique to the individual body—if you have any concerns you should seek advice from your doctor.

Healthy nutrition

It is not healthy for women to diet until they are very thin. If your body doesn't get proper nourishment, this will negatively affect your mood and energy levels, and can cause long-term health problems such as fertility troubles, heart disease, and bone thinning.

This is not to say that all-you-can-eat buffets and extra-large fries are healthy either. Excess weight affects your self-esteem and fitness level, and can damage your sex life. When unhealthy, fatty, sugary foods are coupled with a lack of exercise, you have a perfect recipe for an unsatisfactory sex life—especially if your partner is leading an equally unhealthy lifestyle.

The power of sex

When something goes wrong in the bedroom, for example, when a woman's sexual response decreases or her pleasure levels off, she may often dismiss her situation as unfortunate, but not life-threatening. But all the body's functions are inherently linked, so if something goes awry in the bedroom, there is a chance it might be an early warning sign of other physical problems. In men, for example, erectile dysfunction is often one of the first warning signs of poor blood flow and decreased circulation.

By listening to our bodies, we can address problems early on and prevent health problems from developing into dangerous conditions. A healthy sex life is an important part of a healthy body, so denying yourself the opportunity to enjoy your sex life to the full does not just cheat you out of pleasure, it cheats you out of a full, happy life. Both your sex life and your overall quality of life will benefit greatly if you become knowledgeable about your body and your partner's body.

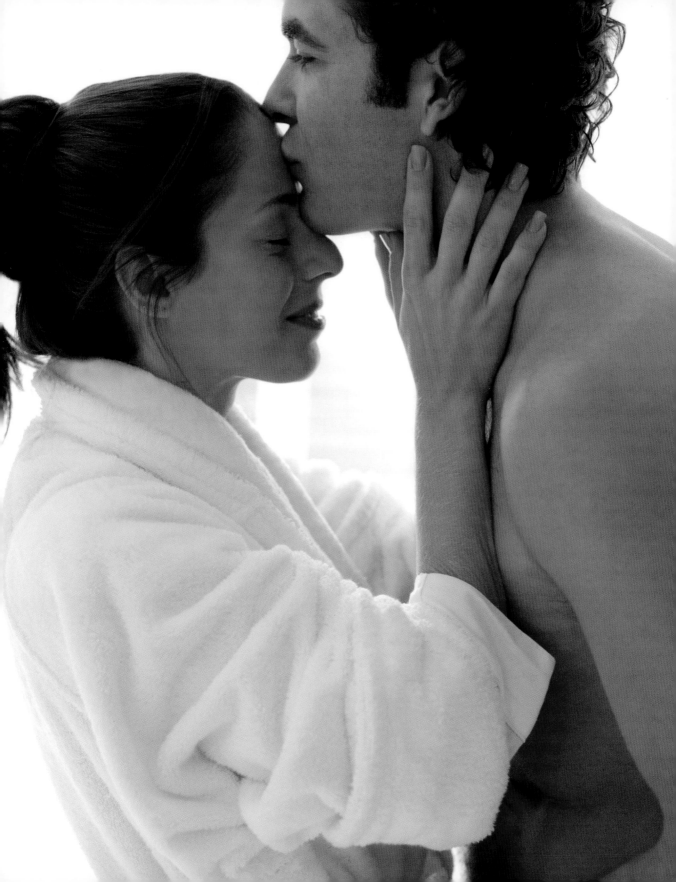

Health and nutrition

We all know that eating an apple is better than eating a donut, walking is healthier than driving, and taking the stairs is better than taking the elevator. But knowing the healthy choice isn't the same as making it—we need motivation. A motivating factor might be that your sex life will benefit enormously from toned muscles and increased stamina. Getting fit for sex doesn't have to be tortuous—in fact, an all-night session with your lover counts as great exercise.

Eating for sex

Too many carbohydrates makes for poorly sexed couples. This doesn't mean you have to cut out carbohydrates—just try to monitor how many and what type you are eating. The more simple sugars you eat, such as those in white bread and cakes, the more insulin your body has to produce. Insulin causes the body to store fat, and it also increases levels of cortisol (the "stress hormone"). Replace simple sugars with complex carbohydrates, such as wholewheat bread and wholegrain pasta. This simple diet change can make a difference to your health, mood, and sex drive.

Date night

For many people, a night of romance often begins with a special meal and a few drinks at their favorite restaurant. But even though you think you are setting the mood for romance, beware. When people eat out in restaurants, they often eat hundreds more calories than they would at home. Larger portion sizes, too much carbohydrate, and alcohol create lethargic, stuffed couples—not a good way to start off a sexy evening for the two of you. Cut back on the calorie overload by avoiding the bread basket and sharing a dessert with your partner. Eat and drink lightly, and you will be hungry for sex when you make it home.

Drink up

We all know the benefits of a nutritious, healthy diet, but water is nature's life-giver. The more water you drink, the more hydrated your system will be and the better your metabolism will work. Our bodies need water to keep our digestive tract in good order; water also helps keep hunger

Your sex life will benefit from regular exercise, and the endorphin rush will create a more relaxed, sexed-up, and happy you.

pangs at bay. Keeping your body hydrated during exercise is also important. If you aren't a plain-water fan, try drinking flavored water or water with a slice of lemon. This simple, painless choice can help you stay fit and healthy, and can keep your skin looking beautiful, too.

Cardiovascular exercise

If you want to reap the amazing benefits of regular exercise—such as improved mood, increased cardiovascular health, and a smaller waistline—you need to get your heart rate up for 30 minutes, three to five times a week. You can get this exercise in a number of fun ways. Walk briskly around the neighborhood, walk or bike to work a few times a week, challenge your partner or the kids to a game of volleyball or soccer, or put on a CD and dance. Committing to an exercise program isn't easy, especially if you hate the activity, so find something you love to do. Your sex life will benefit, and the endorphin rush will create a more relaxed, sexed-up, and happy you.

Sexercise

Some types of exercise are beneficial to your overall health, some prepare you to run a marathon, and some make you look good in a swimsuit. Sexercise is exercise that gets you in tune with your sexual side.

Many cities now offer dance classes such as salsa and pole-dancing. These classes increase your heart rate and tone your muscles. Dancing will also put you in touch with your wild, sexy side.

Yoga is a great part of a sexercise routine as it improves your muscle tone and core strength. Strong muscles and stamina mean new sex positions and renewed strength in old ones.

Sexercise can be anything that gets your body engaged in a sexy way, your muscles moving, and your confidence soaring. Try to do one sexercise workout every week. Remember, a sexy body is a healthy body, so get moving.

Sleeping for sex

Sleep makes you feel refreshed and clear-headed. Adults need six to eight hours of sleep a night. Lack of sleep causes you to eat more and be bad-tempered—not great for your sex life. Try to cut out watching TV before bed. The blue lights from the screen have been shown to disturb sleep patterns. Relaxation exercises can prepare your body and mind for sleep. And an orgasm is the best sleep inducer of all.

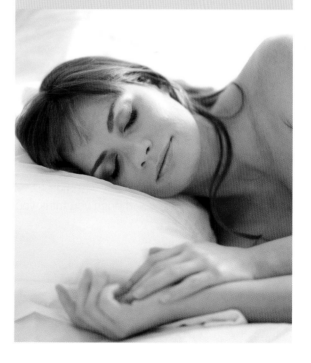

Sex during pregnancy

Conception and pregnancy can be the most beautiful events in any relationship, but they also present unique challenges in the bedroom. Shifting hormones, feelings of exhaustion or nausea—or both—an ever-changing body, worries about forthcoming labor, and the looming responsibilities of parenthood can all hinder sex drive for men and women. It is not surprising that the prospect of staying sexy during the nine months might seem a little daunting.

Before pregnancy
Not everyone plans to get pregnant, but a little forward planning creates the best possible conditions for you and your partner to conceive.

Poor diet and lifestyle have been linked to male and female fertility problems. Attaining a healthy weight, eating a diet of fresh organic foods, and avoiding alcohol and tobacco will all improve your chances of getting pregnant.

A check-up with your doctor is also a good idea, so you can talk over health concerns or discuss the effects of any prescription medication on your or your partner's fertility. Women are also advised to take 400 micrograms of folic acid daily before conception and for the first three months of pregnancy to assist healthy neural development in the baby. Men might find a zinc and vitamin supplement helpful in boosting their fertility.

Getting pregnant
Sometimes, even talking about getting pregnant can put the brakes on your sex life. Starting a family is a wonderful thing to do, but it is not a sexy topic of conversation. This is particularly true if, after several months or more of trying, you both start to feel stressed about not conceiving.

Couples are usually advised to have sex three or four times during the woman's fertile time. But this can feel very unsexy if neither of you is in the mood for lovemaking. You have a common goal—having a baby—so don't worry if sex during this time feels functional rather than fun. This is fine as long as the rest of the time your sex life is as sexy and wild as you want it to be.

Safe sex during pregnancy
Sex during pregnancy is safe most of the time. If you are having a "normal" pregnancy, your doctor will tell you to enjoy your sex life. However, you may be advised to abstain from sex if you are diagnosed as having a high-risk pregnancy. This might include, but is not limited to, conditions such as placenta previa or cervical incompetence.

Avoiding sex may also be advised if you are having any unexplained vaginal bleeding. Sometimes doctors warn mothers pregnant with twins (or more) not to have sex near the end of their pregnancy, due to fear of preterm labor. In fact, if you are at risk of preterm labor for any reason, your doctor might advise avoiding sex, since prostaglandins in semen can cause your body to have contractions.

As far as foreplay goes, continue your usual routine, with one caveat: remind your partner not to blow air into your vagina. This can cause a potentially fatal air embolism in the baby. Instead, tell him to rely on tongue and finger techniques.

Nine sexy months

Just because you are pregnant doesn't mean you can't look sexy. Put financial worries aside and purchase some sexy maternity clothes, bras, and panties. Your body will appreciate their tailor-made support, you will feel attractive, and your partner will love the effect of lace on your blooming figure. Enjoy your body. This is one time in your life when big is allowed to be beautiful.

For this reason, women often find pregnancy to be a time of sexual intimacy with their lover. As the body prepares for childbirth, some women experience heightened libido caused by an increase in vaginal lubrication and genital blood flow, leading to a hypersensitive clitoris.

You might be in the mood for sex but find your changing shape means your favorite position is uncomfortable. Most couples find that side-by-side positions are perfect since they keep the weight off the woman's belly and allow her to control the thrusting. Woman-on-top positions are also comfortable and sexy—particularly if your partner is turned on by your peach- or pear-shaped belly. The only positions to avoid are ones that put you flat on your back, as this decreases your blood circulation and poses a risk to your baby.

Your baby may sometimes respond to your orgasm by waking up and kicking, or be lulled to sleep by the motions of your lovemaking. Both reactions are normal but—as always—report any significant or prolonged changes in your baby's activity to your doctor or midwife promptly.

As D-day approaches, take advantage of your time alone before the little bundle arrives. You might not have the opportunity—or energy—for spontaneous sex for quite some time.

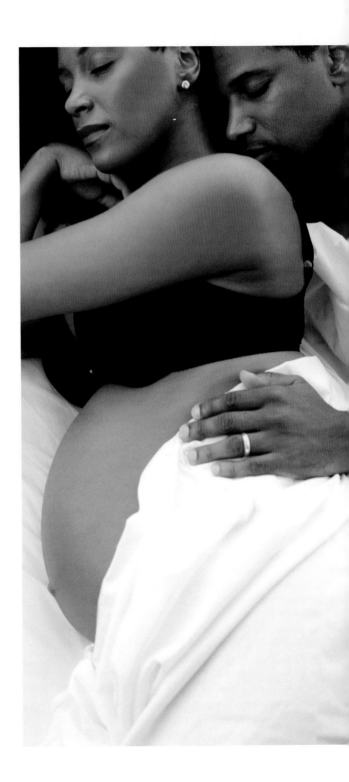

Sex during menopause

Men and women sometimes struggle to maintain a happy, healthy sex life during the so-called "change of life." Menopause and andropause (male menopause) can disrupt your hormones, mood, libido, and relationship—changes for which many couples are not prepared. Physical changes often coincide with emotional upheavals, such as your children leaving home, retirement, and concerns about aging, adding to your burden. However, surviving this difficult time with your sex life strong and intact is possible.

Menopausal symptoms
The menopause is the natural stopping of a woman's monthly periods. The drop in hormones that comes with it brings many unpleasant symptoms—hot flashes, insomnia, weight gain, mood swings, and vaginal dryness, to name just a few—which can create low libido and negatively affect a women's sexual enjoyment. Fortunately, all of these symptoms can be treated.

Simple home remedies
The depletion of estrogen can throw your sleeping habits out of whack, and you will feel the effects of it in all areas of your life, including your sex life. To overcome this, practice good nocturnal habits. Go to bed at the same time every night and wake at the same time every morning, including on the weekends. This keeps your body's natural rhythm intact. Try herbal remedies such as chamomile tea before bed, or spraying lavender water on your pillow at night.

More than 75 percent of women suffer from hot flashes during menopause. Hot flashes occur when a dip in estrogen levels causes stellate ganglion nerves—the part of the brain responsible for body temperature regulation—to work overtime. Although there is no cure, they can be treated with a few behavioral remedies, which will help you get back in the mood for sex.

During the day, dress in cool, cotton fabrics, and keep moist wipes and a miniature fan in your handbag. A fan in the bedroom will keep you cool while you make love. You can also keep a bowl of cool water by the bed. When you feel hot, put your feet in the bowl—this lowers your body temperature and offers instant relief.

Talk with your partner about your needs. If menopausal symptoms cause you to need more foreplay, lubrication, or stimulation to get in the mood for sex, speak up and ask for what you want. Your partner will appreciate your directness.

Hormonal help
Hormonal imbalance also causes low libido, a common menopausal complaint. Your doctor can assess your levels of estrogen, progesterone, and testosterone. If you have a hormonal imbalance, topical hormones in the form of gels, creams, and patches can help. Hormones that enter your body through your skin are preferable to those that are taken orally, because they don't circulate through your body to the same extent.

Hormone Replacement Therapy (HRT) can also be an effective treatment for menopausal symptoms. If you are concerned about the link between HRT and increased risk of stroke, heart disease, and breast cancer, speak to your doctor. Don't dismiss HRT as a treatment option—your doctor will be able to give you individually tailored advice about what is best for you.

Getting back in the mood for sex
Sex during this time can keep you feeling healthy and fit. Being intimate with your partner will keep your relationship strong and keep you in touch with your sensual feminine side.

Good circulation and lubrication are both important to maintain sexual health. Prescription drugs can help women overcome a flagging sexual response, but there are also a number of natural methods that can improve desire.

Dancing, walking, and jogging improve blood circulation and prime your body for sex. The genital tissues thin out as you age, so lubrication is important, too. Warming lubricants will give a pleasurable tingle to your genitals. And a vibrator is helpful in improving sexual desire. Experiment with new positions and techniques—it might give you and your man the incentive to discover your sex life all over again.

Supporting your partner
If you or your partner need prescription medication to boost your libido or treat a hormonal imbalance, this can be an added bonus for both of you in the bedroom. In fact, when one partner gets libido treatment, the other partner's sexual response and libido improve, too. This is due to the fact that having more sex inevitably drives the desire and arousal of both partners.

Give and ask for loving support throughout the menopausal years. If either of you needs to go to the doctor, go to appointments together—good sexual health can be a team effort.

Andropause
Men often suffer a depletion of testosterone as they age, which causes symptoms such as low energy, insomnia, erectile dysfunction, weight gain, and low libido. Treatments for andropause usually include Testosterone Replacement Therapy (TRT) in the form of injections, pills, or creams to stabilize testosterone levels. TRT is a viable treatment for most men, but is unsuitable for those with prostrate cancer, because the testosterone may cause the cancer to spread or grow. If your partner is suffering mainly from erectile dysfunction, prescription drugs can help improve blood flow to the genitals and give him stronger erections. However, men with heart conditions or those taking nitrates should not take certain medications. Encourage your partner to talk through his options with a doctor to find the best treatment for his symptoms.

Sex during later life

Just because you and your partner are older doesn't mean you can't enjoy a rich and rewarding sex life. Older lovers don't have the same sex worries as younger couples, such as pregnancy, work pressure, and childcare. Use this time to rediscover the adventure in your sex life. Spend your days having sex where and how you want it. Hold hands in the kitchen, run naked through the house, and enjoy the cool breeze while making love in the garden. Think of it as a new beginning for your relationship.

New freedoms

Despite what you might think to the contrary, you are never too old for sex. Being older has its advantages. You have more time and more patience. In fact, more than 50 percent of people aged 65–74 are still sexually active, while 25 percent of people aged 75–85 still enjoy sexual activity. There is really is no such thing as being too old—as long as your body is on board.

Sex after your 60th birthday can be liberating. For one thing, unwanted pregnancy is no longer an issue. For another, most men and women at that age have reached an acceptance of their bodies that younger men and women cannot relate to. Life lessons bring the overall realization that wrinkles, curves, and cellulite are part of the beauty of sex, helping to create a love life that is refreshingly free of body-image woes.

Stay sexy

Just because you are older doesn't mean you can look and feel sexy. Invest in sensual lingerie in flattering colors and in materials such as silk or satin that feel good against your skin. Treat yourself and your partner to regular massage and spa appointments—both of these activities improve your overall feeling of health and well-being, and improve blood flow and sexual desire. Weekends away and vacations alone with your partner also keep your relationship feeling special. Warm climates, comfortable hotel rooms, and a change of scene can do wonders for helping you to reconnect with each other and get back in the mood for sex.

Changes to sexuality

You might notice a change in your genitals as you get older. As men and women change and age, so do their sexual organs. You may notice differences in the sensations of sex. As women age, the vagina shortens and narrows, and vaginal lubrication often decreases. As a result, you might need to rely on over-the-counter lubrications more than you previously did. Choose a water-soluble lubricant or experiment with one with a warming sensation to spice up your foreplay.

Your partner's genitals may also change with age. Many men encounter erectile dysfunction in some form by the age of 65. Your partner might feel his erections are not as hard or as large as they used to be, and it might take him longer to become aroused.

Prescription drugs can improve your partner's erections and help you to become aroused, but they can't create desire or intimacy. If you and your partner have other sexual concerns—such as wanting sex to be more exciting—you will need to address them alongside the medication.

Circulation is the main obstacle for older couples wanting to attain a satisfying sex life. This means that exercise and a healthy lifestyle are crucial in keeping you and your partner fit for sex. You don't have to join a gym—activities such as gardening, walking, dancing, swimming, and playing with your grandchildren all get your blood moving and count as good exercise.

Other physical changes

Aging can lead to joint pain, rheumatism, and arthritis, which can create pain during certain sex positions or make it difficult to maintain physical activity for long periods of time. Try taking a warm bath before sex, and keep your bedroom warm so you can dispense with heavy blankets and quilts.

Spend plenty of time on foreplay, such as erotic massage, to prime your responses before having sex. Use positions that avoid pressure on your joints—such as missionary, spooning, or seated positions—and, when you feel discomfort, use it as an opportunity to keep things exciting and change into another position.

Healthy activity

Older women benefit from masturbation, even if they have never done it before. Self-stimulation reduces the thinning and drying of the vagina— vaginal atrophy—that naturally occurs in older women, and it also improves your physical and emotional mood. This is true even if you have heart disease and worry that the physical stress of sex may put you at risk of a heart attack.

Provided your doctor has approved sex, and you want to continue having it, then there is truly no such thing as a "sexpiration" date.

The first time, again

Dating and intimacy after the death of your spouse might feel like a betrayal. You need time to recover and grieve for your loved one before starting a new relationship. After years of making love with one person, you might find you are out of practice when it comes to having sex with a new man. Share your feelings with him— he is probably as nervous as you are. Practice safe sex, even if there is no risk of pregnancy.

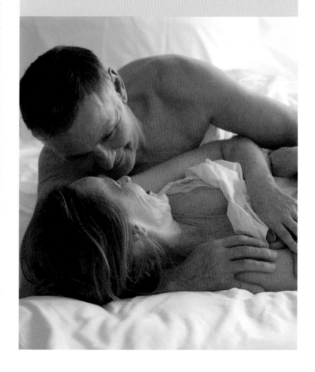

Sex files: Sex after sixty

Remaining sexually active in later life is a great way to stay emotionally and romantically bonded with your partner. It also keeps you feeling young, sexy, and vibrant. This is how one couple revived their sex life, despite health problems and a belief that people over the age of 60 "don't have sex."

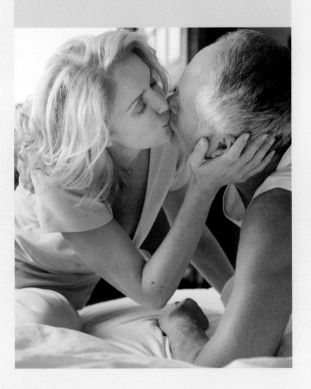

Background

Martin, 60 years old, and Victoria, 62 years old, have been married for 11 years. They have a close relationship and have supported each other through illness—Martin has diabetes and back problems, and Victoria had breast cancer, which she has just recently recovered from.

The problem

Victoria's sex drive waned considerably after she was diagnosed with breast cancer, and didn't return when she got better. This, plus the fact that they both had busy lives helping out with grandchildren, meant they hadn't had sex in almost three years. Despite an otherwise happy relationship, Martin and Victoria were growing irritable and impatient with each other. Martin was keen to resume his sex life with Victoria, although he said he sometimes found it difficult to maintain an erection. Victoria's response to Martin's request for sex was, "I'm over 60. Who has sex in their 60s?"

Finding solutions

After assuring Victoria and Martin that many people have active sex lives well into their 60s, 70s, and beyond, I recommended that they make physical health a priority. This included healthy eating (which is of special importance for Martin because he has diabetes), daily exercise, and regular check-ups with their doctors. I reminded them that the more frequently people have sex, the more they want and enjoy it, and the more able their bodies respond sexually.

Next, I proposed a five-step plan to help them rebuild their sex life. The first step was to restore intimacy (and counteract impatience and irritability) by bringing back neglected tokens of affection: I asked them to use pet names for each other, buy each other little gifts, and cuddle and kiss.

The second step was for Victoria to start giving herself "me" time. I wanted her to stop focusing exclusively on her grandchildren so that she could get out of her "grandma" mindset and rediscover herself as a woman. To help this process I asked her to buy a simple, no-frills clitoral vibrator to re-awaken her sexual responses.

Thirdly, I asked Victoria and Martin to spend time naked in bed stroking and massaging each other. This hopefully would get them interacting sexually again, with the benefit that prolonged caressing would give Victoria the chance to lubricate and Martin the chance to get a firm erection.

The fourth step was to look at erotica together—either print or film. This would boost both Martin's and Victoria's arousal levels and increase their chance of orgasm.

Finally, I asked Victoria and Martin to try a new sex position. Instead of the missionary position—always their favorite in the past—I asked Martin to try sitting on the bed or sofa and to get Victoria to sit on his lap. This would not only prevent back pain for Martin, but would allow Victoria to control the rhythm, speed, and depth of penetration.

What happened?

Martin and Victoria tried all of the steps I recommended—as a result they started cuddling, caressing, and being playful with each other again. In time this also led to sex. Martin said he found it extremely arousing to look at erotica with Victoria. She, in turn, loved the vibrator: "One night with it and I felt like a new woman."

Resist stereotypes

If you're over 60, don't buy into the myth that you can't have a fulfilling sex life. Let yourself be led by your sex drive and desires. If you have health problems that impact on sex, there are plenty of drugs and treatment options available. Ask your doctor for advice.

A healthy mind

Good mental health is important for good sex. If we are relaxed, self-confident, and positive, these attributes will be reflected in our sex lives. But if we are stressed, self-conscious, and burdened with negative thoughts about our body or relationships—or even just life in general—the chances are that sex will suffer. If some aspect of your sex life isn't working, it may be your mind rather than your body that needs attention. Fortunately, there are many ways to start feeling good about yourself.

Positive thinking

Being positive about ourselves and the people we love is vital to creating a healthy mind. Too often our thoughts are composed of terms such as "I can't" and "I'm not." Once you banish these types of negative thoughts, you will have room for more positive ones. Instead of "I hate my thighs. I need to lose weight," try thinking, "I have a plan to get into shape." The first thought cuts you down and makes you feel negative about yourself while the second empowers you and builds you up. The two thoughts are both focused on the same goal—becoming fit—but their results are likely to be very different.

As simple as it might sound, the best way to create a healthy mind is to love yourself more. If you are kind to yourself, you can prevent negative thoughts from taking over your mind, and stop yourself getting caught up in negative emotions.

A useful exercise is to write down your negative thoughts or experiences on pieces of paper, then burn them or throw them away. As you burn the paper, you might find that the metaphor becomes literal, and that as each piece of paper burns and sizzles, the very thoughts in your brain lose their power over you.

Accepting your sexual past

If inhibitions are preventing you from enjoying your sex life, try this exercise: Identify your negative thoughts and beliefs about your sexuality, and sex in general. Write them down on little slips of paper. Look at each slip of paper and ask yourself: Where did this message come from? Who taught it to me? Is it true? Can I create new rules for myself? Once you figure out what prevents you from enjoying your sex life to the full, you can better address the negative thoughts and create a healthy mindset, both inside and outside the bedroom.

Mind therapy

Throughout your life you will probably experience the full spectrum of emotions: incredible joy when you succeed; anger and frustration when you fail; periods of stress, anxiety, and worry; intense grief when you lose a loved one; and happiness when you find a new love. Often we don't know how to manage the negative and positive emotions that occur naturally in our day-to-day lives. Life is a delicate balancing act, but keeping your mind healthy and your sex life intact makes it much easier to manage life's ups and downs.

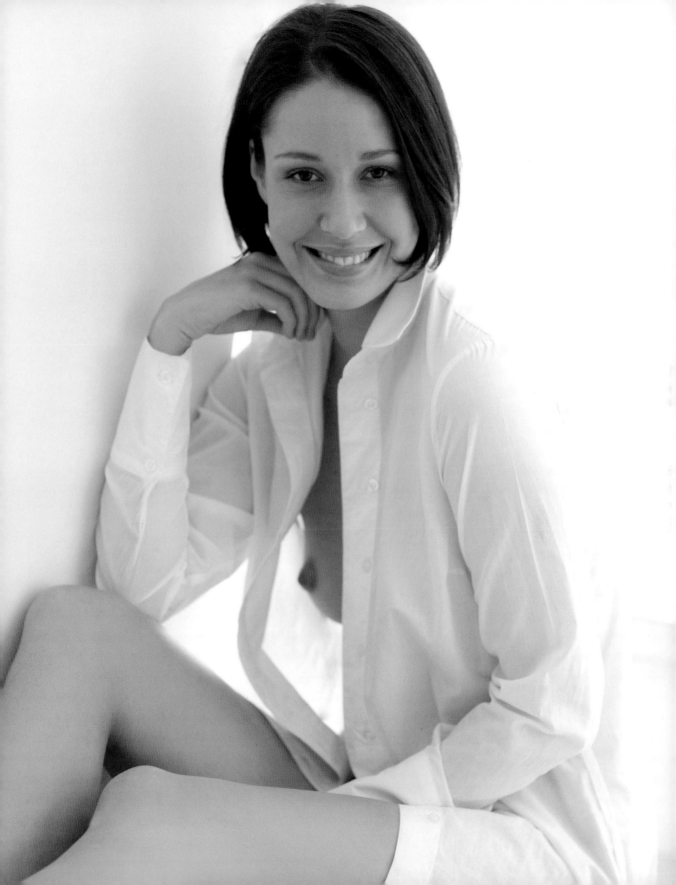

Sex and stress

It is impossible to avoid stress—it's everywhere. Unmanaged stress, whatever its source, creates a cocktail of unpleasant symptoms, from nervous anxiety, insomnia, and indecisiveness to indigestion, muscle tension, and skin rashes. It is a bona fide libido killer. But you can learn to utilize stress as a motivator when necessary, and then decrease it when you want to relax—when you are at home in bed, for example—helping you to survive any hellish week, or month, for that matter.

The purpose of stress

In small doses, stress can be useful in dealing with high-pressure situations, such as sitting an exam, giving a presentation, or winning a race. In these circumstances, it can also be conducive to a good sex life. However, long-term stress caused by life-altering events, such as moving house or planning a big event like a wedding, can leave you feeling permanently frazzled. Cope with stress by putting it into perspective. In other words, unless the situation is life-threatening, don't let stressful events overtake all areas of your life.

Sexual response to stress

Men and women tend to respond differently to stress. Stress tends to make women feel moody and exhausted, whereas your man might have one thing on his brain: sex. When men are under stress, the hormones in their bodies prompt the fight-or-flight response, which increases testosterone production. This was important for our ancestors, as it helped them to fight off danger (in the form of wild animals, for example) or flee from it. And men still experience the same adrenalin-pumping reaction to stress when confronted with a less toothy, but still stressful situation, such as an angry boss. So don't be surprised when your partner comes home randy and ready after a hard day at work.

You might know from experience that you don't feel this same sexual energy after a bad day at the office. This is because women respond to stress by going into a tend-and-befriend mode. When confronted with danger, our female ancestors had to protect their children (tend) and rely on other women for support (befriend).

After a bad day, many women respond by calling up a girlfriend or female family member to talk over the situation. At one time, this female sharing of information may have helped women survive potentially dangerous situations.

This response is great for our friendships, but it is not so great for our sex lives. When women are stressed, their bodies release oxytocin, which leads to a decrease of free circulating testosterone in the body. And this hormonal chain reaction leaves women less physiologically primed for sex.

Overcoming your stress

To prevent stress from completely overtaking your sex life, set aside a quiet time every night. Sometimes all you need to get back into a positive, confident frame of mind is 15 to 30 minutes by yourself. Ask your partner to watch the kids for a while (trade roles after your quiet time so he also has time to himself) and engage in a relaxing activity—think long bath, hot shower, or yoga. Use your time wisely and engage in whatever activity calms you down and takes you from feeling stressed to sexy and relaxed.

If you can fit it into your schedule, then 30 minutes of cardiovascular exercise can help you cope with stress at home or the office. Visiting the gym after work will also give you some much-needed space to get over your day before heading home. If your schedule or home life make this difficult, take mini-breaks throughout the day—such as a quick walk around the block or a quiet cup of tea sitting in the garden—in order to keep yourself from going into overdrive.

Combatting stress together
The best way to maintain a healthy work/life balance is to maintain a healthy balance in your relationship as well. If you are feeling stressed and anxious and are harboring anger that your partner is not pulling his weight, you will have a recipe for tension and arguments.

Try to bring a little humor into your life. Watch a funny movie together, put on a favorite CD and dance, or spend some time chasing a ball around the garden with your children. Do whatever it takes to change the mood from stress and tension to a more fun and relaxing atmosphere.

Take turns nurturing each other. When one person is having a bad week at work, for example, the other could make a commitment to cook dinner or put the kids to bed. A healthy relationship is based on give-and-take.

Even if you don't initially feel like having sex when you come home after a hard day, being intimate with your man rather than starting a fight with him may awaken your sexual desire. And an orgasm will defeat stress every time.

Mind space

Meditation can teach you to still your mind and focus on the present, so joining a yoga class can be helpful in managing stress. Breath and body control combine to leave you feeling calmer and more rational. And any activity that distances you from domestic, work, or other stress is helpful in keeping you focused on the important things in life, such as your well-being and your relationships with your loved ones.

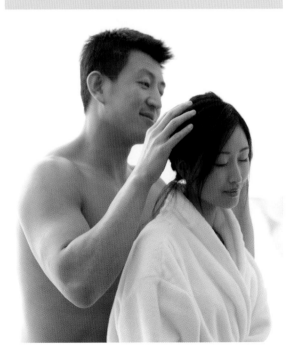

Sex and emotional distress

Our emotions affect more than just our mood. They affect our physical and sexual health, along with our relationships. Often we don't know how to manage negative emotions, which are a natural result of our day-to-day lives. Sadness caused by the loss of a loved one, everyday worry and anxiety, and feelings of anger toward a partner can all have a detrimental effect on sex. However, finding positive ways to deal with your distress can help to keep a sexual and emotional connection alive in your relationship.

Sex during times of grief

Whether you are dealing with the death of a loved one, the end of a relationship, or another cause of grief, loss is difficult to come to terms with, and causes a range of distressing symptoms, such as insomnia, anxiety, restlessness, changes in appetite, and depression. When you don't feel like getting out of bed in the morning, it can be difficult to be in the mood for any sort of intimacy and this can affect your relationship.

For some couples, sex can help. Making love allows a couple to return, albeit briefly, to a semblance of feeling normal, provided that each partner is allowed to take their time and decide whether sex feels right in the current situation. Sex can be comforting—it can offer a welcome respite from a trying time and temporarily relieve distress, and can make you feel more in control.

If neither of you is up to making love during this time, keep your bond strong by maintaining touch and intimacy. If you don't maintain some affection, the lack of physical contact may create a lack of emotional intimacy as well. Take baths together, give each other back rubs, or just lie in the spoons position in bed. Sometimes just having a good cry can help keep your relationship strong—and give you both emotional catharsis. If you are having trouble caring for yourself, then having another person to take care of you can make all the difference to your recovery time.

Sex during the healing process

Grief, like any serious illness, needs to run its course. It can take several years to come to terms with grief, particularly if a bereavement occurs in tragic or untimely circumstances. However, most

Making love allows a couple to return, albeit briefly, to a semblance of normality. Keep your bond strong by maintaining touch and intimacy.

people recover, and naturally and gradually accept their loss with time. For those who become stuck in a grief cycle, it can help to see a trained therapist. A therapist will not only help you come to terms with your loss but can help you stay emotionally open with your partner—this will make it easier for you to stay sexually intimate.

Sex during times of anger

Most couples have fights and disagreements. It doesn't mean they can't work through their problems, but anger can have a damaging effect on a couple's sex life.

Pinpointing the causes of anger in a relationship isn't always easy. Sometimes we confuse anger with other emotions, such as frustration, hurt, or sadness. You might discover the reason you thought you were angry had nothing to do with the real reasons. For example, you might think you are angry with your partner for not spending enough time with you, but the real reason for your anger may be a change in your career or other circumstances that have caused you to spend more time alone. Discovering the reason for tension and anger in a relationship is always the first step in resolution.

If neither of you is willing to make a truce, then agree not to be intimate during this time. Anger is not good for your nervous system or for your relationship, so agree to disagree for the time being. If arguments and disputes are ongoing, consider seeing a couples' therapist, who can help you both work through your conflict.

However, if you are both willing to stay intimate through times of conflict, try experimenting sexually—use new positions and techniques to break out of your previous relationship script. Sex and intimacy can help you to stay connected during a rocky patch. A close, sexual bond can also help to heal your relationship. All couples get angry, but if you make him sleep on the couch, you might be setting yourself up for a longer fight.

Sex when you're sad

Common causes of emotional distress, such as health or relationship problems, can zap sexual energy and interest. However, sex can be exactly what you need—the endorphins released during sex are natural relaxants and mood-enhancers. If you can't muster the energy for sex, talk about your feelings to your partner, or to a friend or therapist. Your libido will return as you learn new ways to cope with difficult feelings.

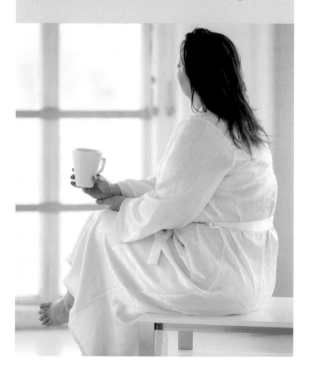

Sex and depression

One of the main symptoms of depression is a loss of interest in things you once loved, and this might include sex and the relationship with a loved one. Many women suffering from depression also experience a loss of interest in their health, grooming, and relationships, all of which can add up to a lack of intimacy. Research also points to a relationship between sexual dysfunction—such as low libido—and depression, although it is uncertain which comes first, the depression or dysfunction.

Symptoms of depression
Depression is a word that gets tossed around a lot, so it can be hard to know if you or your partner are suffering from clinical depression or are just feeling a little blue. Symptoms vary but generally people suffering depression report one or all of the following: feeling lost, helpless, or hopeless; sleep or appetite changes; loss of energy, concentration, motivation, and interest in daily activities; irritability; and self-loathing. If you or your partner are experiencing these feelings on a daily basis, seek help from a medical professional immediately.

Whether or not to have sex
Sex can be an important part of overcoming depression, thanks to endorphins, which flood your brain during orgasm. But choosing whether to have sex or to abstain is a tricky decision. It is often recommended that when a person is recovering from depression, addiction, or other serious emotional disturbances, they should not date or be physical with other people during their recovery process. Many people suffering from depression feel they need time and emotional space to heal their mind before starting to have regular sex again. This is particularly true if you are struggling with low libido or if you are not emotionally ready for intercourse during this time.

You can stay intimate and connected to your partner by being loving and affectionate with him—reach out for emotional connection with him. Your decision to have sex or not is one that you need to make with your partner and your doctor. Whatever your decision, your mental health and well-being should be given priority.

Stay intimate with and connected to your partner by being loving and affectionate with him— reach out for emotional connection with him.

Unhealthy sex

Regardless of which comes first for an individual—depression due to lack of sexual interest and activity or vice versa—we know that the two are inherently connected.

Although depression can negatively affect your sex drive, this connection doesn't always lead to a lack of sex. A mild to a moderately depressed woman is likely to have sex more often than a woman who is not depressed, to be sexually adventurous, and to engage in casual sex.

Low self-esteem is a common by-product of depression and can lead women to seek sex as a way to counteract negative feelings. Being promiscuous or having casual sex might be self-destructive behavior or a way to find love and acceptance, but it is not emotionally healthy sex.

Talking it through

Women often feel a need to be people-pleasers and present a happy face to the world. As a result, they don't have an outlet for their negative emotions such as fear, self-doubt, and anger. Resolve to find someone you can rely on. Most people suffering from depression choose to speak to a professional therapist, but you might prefer to speak with a religious counselor or faith leader.

Medical treatments

There are many different treatments for depression, including medications that balance the chemicals in the brain. They are not for everyone—and some lead to sexual dysfunction. If you are prescribed medications, don't let potential side effects prevent you from taking the medicine. However, if your doctor has prescribed antidepressants and you are experiencing negative sexual side effects, ask about prescriptions associated with lower rates of sexual side effects. And talk to your doctor about alternative remedies and therapies that might be helpful in overcoming your depression.

Living with depression

Depression can be one of the most difficult struggles to overcome in a person's life, but with the right treatment and care, you can come back from this battle stronger and happier than ever before. Living with a partner with depression can be equally difficult. His condition can affect your mental and physical health, so you need someone to share your feelings with, too. You might feel guilty that you can't do more to help him, and you may also feel frustrated by his illness. Both are normal reactions. Assist his healing process by encouraging him to spend time outdoors with friends and family, reminding him to keep doctor and therapist appointments, and helping him to live a healthy lifestyle. Exercise, regular sleep, and talking will boost his recovery time. Mental and physical support are a crucial step in helping to heal your loved one's body and mind.

A healthy sexual relationship

Before getting intimate with a new partner, your first sexual conversation should be to exchange histories, discuss getting tested, and decide on a method of contraception. These might not be very sensual topics of conversation, but raising them shows that you hold yourself and his health in high esteem. Fulfilling your sexual desires is crucial for your general well-being, but so is maintaining a healthy sex life throughout all stages of your life, even when you are in a long-term relationship.

Healthy sex all of your life

No relationship is complete without the mandatory "sex history" in which new couples share any possible health concerns in their sexual past. This doesn't mean that you have to tell your partner about the one time you had unprotected sex in college, but it does mean that you need to tell him whether or not you have been tested recently (and given a clean bill of health) for all of the major sexually transmitted diseases (STDs).

If neither of you have been tested in a while, it might be a good idea to go together and be each other's support system. It isn't exactly the most romantic discussion you can have with your partner, but it is much better than the discussion you would have to have if one or both of you ended up with an STD.

Contraception

It is a good idea to discuss contraception before you become intimate, but after you know that intimacy is on the cards. In other words, you don't have to discuss your chosen method of contraception on the first date, unless you plan on being intimate with that person right away—but don't wait until you are in the bedroom.

Life with an STD

If you have an incurable STD, such as herpes or HIV, you should tell your partner in a neutral time and place. Don't wait until you are physically intimate. Be prepared for your partner to have questions and concerns—you might want to bring some materials from the internet or your local health clinic that have information for partners who are dating someone with an STD. There are many resources available for couples, so take advantage of the information at your disposal.

Protecting each other

Protection preferences vary from couple to couple, but the most reliable form of protection against STDs is the condom, both for intercourse and when performing oral sex on your partner. When receiving oral sex, women should wear a dental dam to prevent saliva and other fluids from entering their vagina. However, it is important to note that condoms can't completely protect you or your partner from STDs.

Whichever mode of protection you use, the safe-sex talk should be an ongoing part of your relationship with your partner. Keep your and your partner's sexual health a priority.

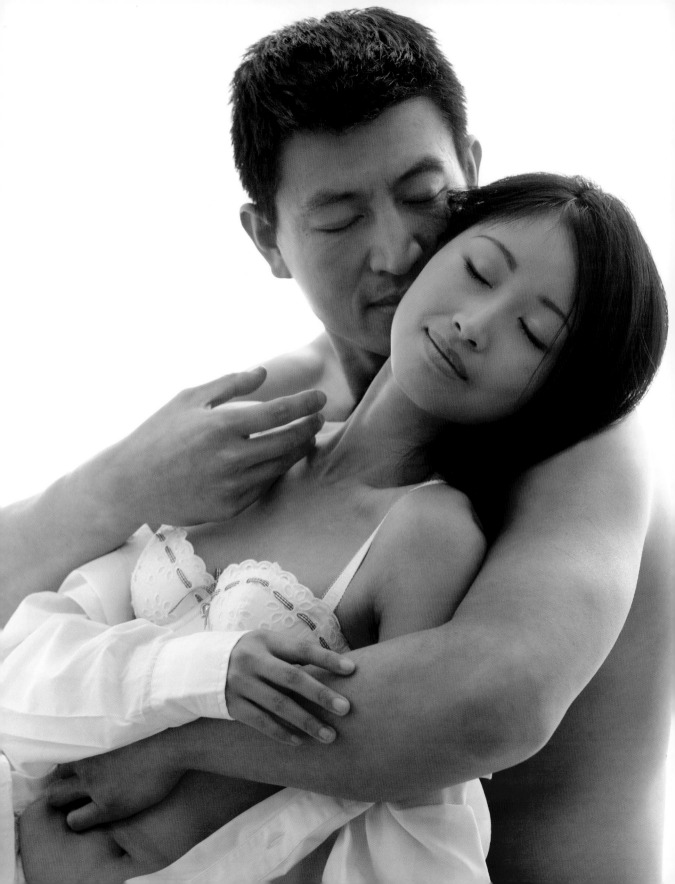

Safer sex

The world is suffering from a veritable epidemic of sexually transmitted diseases (STDs), and practicing safer sex has never been more important. It is vital to educate yourself about STDs and their symptoms, and learn how to protect yourself against them. It is essential for men and women of all ages to understand how to set sexual boundaries, communicate with their partner about their needs for healthy sex, and decide on the protection methods that work best for them.

Educate and protect yourself

To become experts at safer sex, we have to learn how to protect ourselves from transmitting and receiving STDs during all forms of intercourse.

Don't underestimate the negative effects of an STD on your sexuality, your health, and your future relationships. Getting tested for STDs together is a smart way to begin a sexual relationship with a new partner. But all couples, even those in long-term relationships, should make sure that they get tested regularly to warn of any problems.

Human papillomavirus (HPV)

The most common STD is HPV. Left untreated, it can wreak havoc on a woman's reproductive organs, leading to cervical cancer, infertility, and even death. It can also lead to anal cancer in men, although this is very rare. Symptoms include genital warts, which can be flat, raised, or cauliflower-shaped. They can appear on the genitals, anus, or scrotum.

It is a scary fact that most people with HPV never know they have it. The good news is that 90 percent of people who are infected will be cleared of the virus within two years, thanks to the body's immune system. Regular cervical smear tests can detect the virus—or subsequent damage to cervical cells—so that treatment can be given.

An HPV vaccine has also been developed to protect women from four strains of the virus—two of which cause 70 percent of cervical cancer cases, and two of which cause 90 percent of genital warts cases. The HPV vaccine is currently approved for girls aged 9–26, but a vaccine for older women is being researched as well.

Herpes

Herpes is becoming more common, particularly among young people. Unfortunately, there is currently no cure, which means that those who are infected may struggle throughout their lives with the physical symptoms, and with emotional questions such as when and how to tell their sexual partners, as well as what it means for their reproductive health.

Although it is possible to be infected with herpes and never show any symptoms, many people experience at least one breakout—though some people experience breakouts monthly, yearly, or at times of stress. Symptoms include painful sores on the genitals (genital herpes) or mouth (oral herpes). Herpes is transmitted by skin-to-skin contact. You can get genital herpes if your partner has oral herpes and performs oral sex on you, or you can get oral herpes if you perform oral sex on a partner with genital herpes. Once herpes is contracted you are always infectious, even if no sores are visible.

Syphilis

The first stage of syphilis is a sore—called a chancre—on the genitals. The secondary stage is marked by joint pain, muscle aches, a sore throat, flu-like symptoms, patchy hair loss, and a whole-body rash. The only way to protect yourself from contracting syphilis is to use a condom, and even that is not completely foolproof. However, the condition can be treated with penicillin.

Auto-immune deficiency syndrome (AIDS)

Since the AIDS epidemic took hold in the 1980s, there has been much misinformation about the disease. Many myths about HIV persist—for example, that only those in the gay community get infected, or only those who are promiscuous or share needles. Of course, everyone has the potential to be infected with HIV. In fact, 75 percent of women with the virus were infected through heterosexual sex. There is now a range of treatment options available for HIV; if you are affected, your doctor will discuss them with you.

Other common STDs

Chlamydia, gonorrhea, trichomoniasis, and bacterial vaginosis often exhibit similar symptoms, which include a discharge, foul odor, pain, itchiness, or discomfort. Many of these STDs can become more problematic and lead to infertility and other chronic health problems if they are not treated, so it is crucial to see a doctor promptly.

Doctors have seen everything, so never let embarrassment prevent you from seeking medical treatment and asking specific questions.

Sexy safer sex

Male and female condoms mean safer sex, and are a reliable method of protecting yourself and your partner from STDs. You may not think of condoms as sexy, but rolling one down the length of your lover's penis as you sit astride him can be an extremely sensual act. As you smooth it onto his shaft, lean forward to stroke his penis, then lick him from base to tip once he's wearing the condom, as a promise of treats to follow.

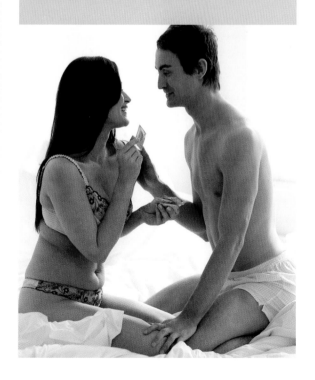

Protection and contraception

Safer sex isn't just important when you are dating casually or in an open relationship. Even those people in long-term relationships should be cautious until they are both given a clean bill of health by a doctor six months after their last unprotected sex session. Most of us will never contract an STD, incurable or otherwise, but it doesn't mean we shouldn't take precautions every time we have sex with every partner. Be smart and safe, and keep your sexual and reproductive health your main priority.

Protecting yourself

Unfortunately, there is no way to protect yourself completely against STDs or unwanted pregnancy, other than abstinence. Any type of skin-to-skin contact, heavy petting, or contact with the genitals can lead to the transmission of viruses. Even manual sex can lead to the spread of bacteria and potentially STDs. For instance, if your partner has a wart on his finger and touches your genitals, you can end up with genital warts.

But oral is safe, right?

Oral sex is sex—it is no less dangerous than intercourse when it comes down to the possible transmission of STDs. Fortunately, there are ways to protect yourself while still enjoying oral sex with your partner, until you are certain that both you and your partner are STD-free.

When performing fellatio, always use a condom. He will still enjoy the sensations of you sucking and licking him, and you will both be safe from the possible spread of infection. Condoms come in different flavors, which might make oral sex more enjoyable for you. Alternatively, when receiving oral sex from your partner, use a dental dam. You place the dental dam over the labia and the opening of the vagina, and this allows your partner to pleasure you without being exposed to vaginal fluids. Plastic wrap can be used for a home-made version, although you must ensure it is free from rips, holes, or tears, and that it covers your genitals completely.

Barrier and hormonal contraceptives

There are plenty of contraceptive choices for couples—IUDs, and hormonal, natural, and barrier methods. Each type comes with risks and benefits, so talk through your options with your doctor or family planning professional.

Barrier methods of contraception prevent the sperm from reaching the fallopian tubes and creating a pregnancy. Two of the most popular barrier methods are condoms and diaphragms. Condoms don't afford much spontaneity and some couples find they detract from the sensation of lovemaking. Regardless, condoms are one of the most effective forms of birth control.

Diaphragms are inserted into the vagina before penetration and create a seal over the cervix, preventing sperm from traveling to the fallopian tubes. Used in conjunction with a spermicide cream or gel, they are about 80 to 85 percent effective in preventing pregnancy. The diaphragm does not affect a couple's enjoyment, although it needs to be used properly to avoid pregnancy, urinary tract infections, and toxic shock syndrome.

IUDs (interuterine devices) are inserted by a doctor and can protect against pregnancy for several years. IUDs operate by disrupting sperm from reaching the egg, and preventing a fertilized egg from implanting in the womb. The benefits are a high degree of protection combined with no sensory or hormonal side affects. However, IUDs can cause heavier periods, and if an IUD slips out of your uterus, you are vulnerable to becoming pregnant.

Hormonal birth control—available as pills, patches, injections, and vaginal rings—is highly effective in preventing pregnancy and often has other benefits as well, such as regulating periods. However, some women suffer from side effects such as low libido, moodiness, or weight gain. For these women, a lower dose of hormonal birth control might help. Since hormonal birth control is highly effective and allows for spontaneity, the benefits may outweigh the side effects.

Natural methods of contraception

Many couples rely on coitus interruptus (where the man withdraws prior to ejaculation), but this method can result in pregnancy. Pre-ejaculate, which is released before a man ejaculates fully, may contain sperm, so the withdrawal method is not advisable as a form of contraception.

Another natural form of contraception is the rhythm method, which is based on a woman's menstrual cycle. During a typical menstrual cycle, a woman has days of fertility (before, during, and after ovulation) when conception is most likely. By abstaining from sex on her "fertile days," a woman can prevent pregnancy. However, this method requires you to know exactly when you ovulate, and the failure rate is up to 25 percent a year, so it is not advisable for all couples.

Sex education

A recent survey in the United States found that one in four teenage girls has an STD, whether it is chlamydia, trichomoniasis, or HPV. This news, combined with soaring rates of teenage pregnancy, underscores the importance of educating young people about sex.

It is easy to blame the media's blatant glamorization of sex, but ignorance and peer pressure also push teenagers into having sex before they are emotionally or physically ready to enjoy it. Teenage girls and boys need more information about STDs, safe sex, and preventing pregnancy. If you have teenage children, try to set a positive example of communication—talk to them about sexual health and encourage their questions. And if you are a teenager, make it your priority to find out the facts about contraception and STDs before you commit to having sex.

Sex addiction

Sex should be a vibrant, exciting, and safe part of every person's life. Unsafe sex may involve being promiscuous or risk-taking, or having sex without protection. Sex addiction is a psychological condition where unusually high sexual activity also becomes emotionally or physically destructive for those involved. Sex addicts don't usually form emotional or intimate bonds with a partner. Addiction is usually progressive, and the key to overcoming it is usually identifying the problem and seeking help.

The dangers of sexual addiction

Sex addiction can mean an addiction to the sex trade, pornography, having sex with strangers, multiple affairs, compulsive masturbation, exhibitionism, voyeurism, obsessive dating, cybersex, sexual harassment, and molestation. More than half of sexual addicts become sex offenders. And the Internet has made it easier for addicts to indulge in a secret and illicit sex life.

Causes and symptoms

A sex addict is defined as a person who is unable to control his or her sexual urges and goes to extreme lengths to fulfill them, no matter what it costs him or her. This means that some people find their entire lives are consumed by seeking the high they receive from sexual activity, even if they are partnered in a long-term relationship.

Behavioral symptoms might include, but are not limited to: excessive flirting or grooming, seeking inappropriate sexual contact, and bartering with sex in exchange for money or power. Addicts often have obsessive thoughts of planning or obtaining sex that intrude upon their personal and work lives—they become distressed if they can't indulge their desires.

The medical profession is unsure why some people are more prone to addiction than others, but there are some factors that sex addicts tend to have in common. Many addicts were sexually abused as children, which leads them to construct unhealthy models for love and pleasure. They also tend to come from dysfunctional families. This can exacerbate a situation of sexual abuse, when the child has no family member to turn to for support.

No sexual behavior is unhealthy unless it becomes a "must" for gratification and gets in the way of intimacy and connection.

Sex addicts are more likely to exhibit addictive behavior in other areas of their lives, and may suffer from alcohol or drug addictions or eating disorders. They are also more likely to have addicts in their families, suggesting that addiction is not just an emotional struggle, but is influenced by genetic factors. Sex addiction is also believed to be associated with other mood and psychological disorders, such as obsessive compulsive disorder (OCD) and depression.

Love addicts

Female addicts are termed "love addicts," because they are not necessarily seeking the high of orgasm in their addictive behavior. Instead, they may seek the euphoria of romance or infatuation that surrounds new sexual encounters.

Symptoms of love addiction are varied but may take the form of a merry-go-round of negative relationships—such as changing relationships and lovers frequently, controlling a lover through sex, and breaking off then returning to an abusive relationship. Love addicts also continue with their behavior despite negative consequences such as broken relationships, shame, remorse, fear, depression, or abuse.

Dangerous sexual behavior

Another damaging form of sexual activity is risky sexual behavior. Bondage and light spanking are quite normal sexual activities. The trouble starts when couples depend on pain as the main source of physical interaction every time they have sex. The regular practice of gagging a submissive partner or inflicting pain or abuse can be physically and emotionally dangerous.

No sexual behaviour is unhealthy unless it becomes a "must" for gratification and gets in the way of intimacy. Communicate with your partner often and openly about your sexual desires. Don't make sexual satisfaction available only through compulsive thrill-seeking.

Getting help

Most addicts don't realize they have a problem, so the first step is to accept their behavior as unhealthy, and then to seek the appropriate help to overcome their problem. Treatment can be complicated by the fact that avoiding sex is not a healthy way to manage sexual feelings either. Cognitive therapy and support groups, which offer online and group sessions, have great success in helping people overcome their addiction. Your doctor can refer you to a trained relationship or pyschosexual therapist, either with or without your partner, depending on your needs. You may also be prescribed psychotherapeutic drugs to help control your moods and obsessive behaviors.

Healing from sex addiction is possible—many people have overcome addiction and created a happy and emotionally healthy sex life for themselves and their partners.

Lust for life: a program

As women of the millennium, our lives are filled with more possibilities than ever before. We can climb the corporate ladder as high it goes, we can start a business, and we can be stay-at-home moms, if we choose to have children at all. Our lives are rich in opportunities. This also means that our lives can be a whirlwind of to-do lists and hectic days and nights. Finding a balance between our love lives—including our sexuality—our roles within our families, and our career goals is the key to happiness.

Live in the present Even if we don't consciously realize it, most of us are waiting for something. We postpone big things like career changes, vacations, heart-to-heart conversations, and continued education, and we postpone small things like learning to cook, starting a new hobby, or losing weight. Our goals get placed on the back burner due to the requirements of our day-to-day lives—with the end result that we can't fully enjoy the present because we are always achieving our goal.

If you want to enhance your sex life and your relationship, I hope this book has helped you begin that journey. From finding ways to discover and communicate your sexual needs, to planning how to incorporate more "me" time into your schedule, I hope you have embraced the "now" philosophy. Now is the time to take that adult-only vacation with your partner, now is the time to sign up for that dance class, and now is the time to act out one of your sexual fantasies. Don't delay the important things—or the fun things—until tomorrow. Enrich your life by making time for them now.

Love your body Living in the present can be difficult if you don't like the way you look. Body image can be one of the major reasons women delay their happiness. A good friend once told me, "Every moment you spend hating your body is a wasted moment of life," and how true this is for many women. Loving our bodies and reaching a "happy weight" sometimes feel like impossible tasks. But the reward of being able to feel good in your own skin is priceless. Whether you make this journey with a friend, your partner, a journal, or a therapist, your growing self-confidence will reshape your life—and be a bright light to the young women who are watching and learning from your steps to a healthy, positive, and realistic body image.

Put yourself first When you board an airplane, the flight attendant reminds you that in the event of an emergency, passengers should put their own oxygen masks on first. Women everywhere need to be reminded of this when it comes to our sexual health and needs. Putting ourselves first isn't easy, especially since women seem raised to think of others before themselves. However, the more you do this, the more you will realize that when you feel happy, healthy, satisfied, and well-rested, the people around you will thrive from your positive presence. Your sexuality is an important part of who you are. If you don't allow it to flourish, you are doing a great disservice to yourself and your loved ones.

Grow with your partner Understanding your partner within the context of your relationship is part of a great sex life. Men and women are equal, but we are still unique when it comes to our thoughts, feelings, hormones, and socialization. These differences are reflected in our relationships and our sex lives—each partner has their own needs in the bedroom. Celebrating these differences and embracing the way they play out in our relationships is the first step in creating great communication and sizzling intimacy.

Embrace your sexuality A great sex life begins with great self-knowledge. From self-love to sexploration with your partner, discovering our own sexual needs is a crucial step on the journey to self-awareness, both sexually and otherwise. By overcoming your inhibitions and championing your own sexuality, you will discover a new-found bravery in all other parts of your life. You will also find deeper intimacy and passion in your relationship with your partner. Here's to breaking out of our uncomfortable cocoons and blossoming into the beautiful, unique, and sexual women that we were born to be.

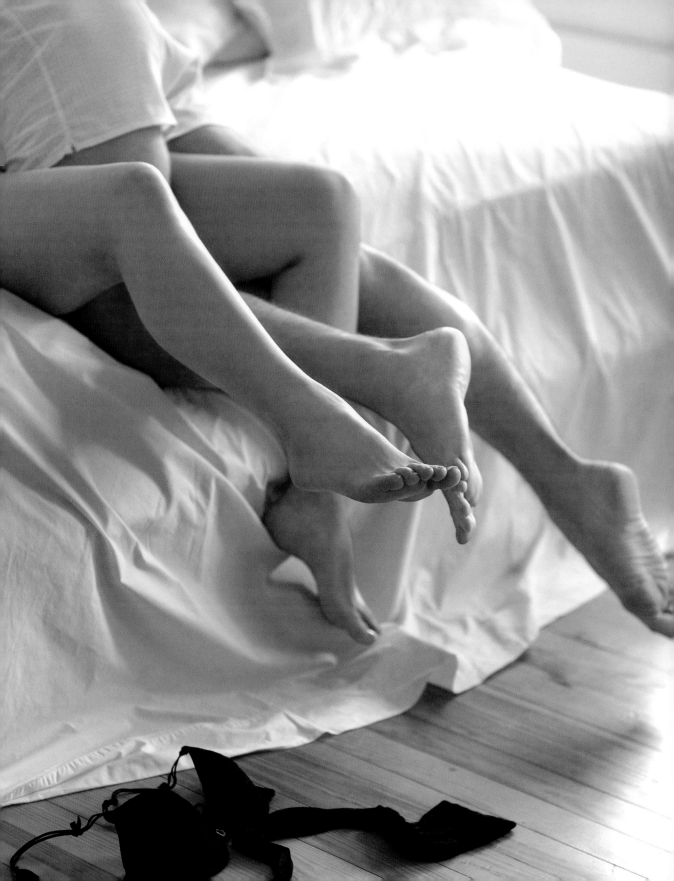

Resources

Creating a vibrant, healthy sex life doesn't happen overnight. Luckily, there are many great resources that women can use to guide them on their journey to fulfilling, joyous sex lives. As you continue to grow and discover your particular sexual tastes and pleasures, these resources can answer your questions, assuage your fears, and help you unleash your inhibitions. From books to websites to erotic toy stores, here is a comprehensive guide to the best sexual health tools for women.

Books

For Women Only
by Jennifer Berman and Laura Berman
(Henry Holt and Company, 2001)
Contains medical information and case studies to help women understand and enjoy their sexuality, with information on drugs, products, and treatments.

Passion Prescription
by Laura Berman
(Hyperion, 2006)
This book is a must-read for all women who want to learn more about their emotional, medical, physical, and social ties to sex.

The Five Love Languages
by Gary Chapman
(Northfield Publishing, 2004)
Like a couples' counseling session, this book shows how to talk and share love with your partner in a way that he or she will understand and give back.

Conscious Loving
by Gay Hendricks and Kathlyn Hendricks
(Bantam, 1990)
Offers tips on communication and relationship agreements, and illustrates how strong commitment in a couple is a byproduct of being a full and complete individual.

Getting the Love You Want
by Harville Hendrix and Helen LaKelly Hunt
(Henry Holt and Company, 2007)
An insightful guide that offers couples techniques for turning criticism and complaints into positive growth and healthy communication.

Guide to Getting it On
by Paul Joannides
(Goofy Foot Press, 2006)
This fun and informative guide covers everything from making out and losing one's virginity to positions and sex toys. It's used in sex ed courses, but it also makes for great erotic reading (either alone, or with a partner!).

Women's Bodies, Women's Wisdom
by Christiane Northrup
(Bantam, 2006)
A holistic approach to women's health within the context of society, family, and work.

How to be a Great Lover
by Lou Paget
(Broadway Books, 1999)
The title doesn't exaggerate! This pithy, informal, and accessible book offers tips (and illustrations) for sex techniques from oral sex to positions.

The Sexy Years
by Suzanne Somers
(Crown, 2004)
A funny, endearing, and practical guide to surviving menopause with your sexiness intact or increasing your sexiness as you age.

The V Book
by Elizabeth G. Stewart and Paula Spencer
(Bantam, 2002)
Informs women about vulvovaginal health, including issues about hygiene and tips for having safe and pleasurable sex.

Kama Sutra For 21st-Century Lovers
by Anne Hooper
(DK Publishing, 2007)
Informs and illustrates, through photos erotic pleasures to arouse and inspire.

Tracy Cox's Kama Sutra
by Tracy Cox
(DK Publishing, 2007)
Photographs and text to illustrate sexual positions inspired by the Kama Sutra and other ancient texts on sex.

Websites

American Association of Sexuality Educators, Counselors, and Therapists
www.aasect.org
804.752.0026
Helps locate a credited sexuality educator, counselor or therapist near you.

The Berman Center
bermancenter.com
800.709.4709
News and appointment-booking for The Berman Center sexual health clinic.

The clitoris.com
www.the-clitoris.com
This educational website is dedicated to the female genitalia, and covers a wide range of topics from anatomy and health to pleasure and sexual function.

Dr. Laura Berman
drlauraberman.com
866.348.7538
Advice and tips on sex and intimacy, including information on sex toys and positions, and details of Dr. Laura Berman products.

National Women's Health Network
www.womenshealthnetwork.org
202.347.1140
Offers health information and vital resources for every woman on all aspects of health, including sex. Also includes the latest health alerts and the Women's Health Activist Newsletter.

The penis.com
www.the-penis.com
A source of useful information about the male genitals. Covers topics from penis size, health and anatomy, to lovemaking and penile massage positions and techniques.

Planned Parenthood
www.plannedparenthood.org
800.230.7526
A comprehensive guide to issues surrounding pregnancy, birth control, STDs, and sexual health. Includes the latest news on reproductive health issues in Washington.

Sex Information and Education Council of the United States
www.siecus.org
A site promoting sexual awareness through sex education and advocacy. It provides detailed information about sexuality and sexual and reproductive health for both adults and adolescents.

Vagina Vérité
vaginaverite.com
A forum for discussing everything vagina-related. The website is dedicated to celebrating a woman's body and sexual exploration.

Shopping

Adam and Eve
adamandevetoys.com
800.293.4654
Sex toys for men and women. Each toy is reviewed and accompanied with tips from users to help you find the perfect toy.

Babeland
www.babeland.com
800.658.9119
Offers all kinds of sex toys, erotica, and sexy gifts. Also gives the locations of Babeland sex toys stores and information on in-store events.

California Exotic Novelties
www.calexotics.com
Offers a wide range of products—from vibrators to lubricants—for everything needed to create mind-blowing sex and fulfill all your fantasies.

Eve's Garden
evesgarden.com/shop
800.848.3837
One of the first proprietors of sex toys for women, Eve's Garden is dedicated to women's sexual pleasure and fun for couples and singles alike.

Good Vibrations
www.goodvibes.com
800.289.8423
Adult products for men and women, including lubricants, books, sex toys, and novelties.

SpicyGear
www.spicygear.com
A woman-owned online store for discreetly packaged sex toys and adult products. Includes reviews and ratings of the items.

Erotica

Femme productions
www.candidaroyalle.com
800.456.5683
A production company that creates pornography with actual storylines and interesting plots, not just sex. Of course, the sex scenes are still racy and highly erotic!

Herotica books
Collections of erotica geared toward women. Great writing combined with adventurous sexual escapades—sure to get your heart racing!

Nancy Friday books
Nancy Friday is the author of various erotica titles. She covers sexual attitudes and fantasies, giving engaging stories of real sexuality.

Index

London, New York, Melbourne, Munich, and Delhi

Editor Nichole Morford
Senior Art Editor Sara Robin
Managing Art Editor Kat Mead
Executive Managing Editor Adèle Hayward
Senior Production Editor Jennifer Murray
US Editor Jane Perlmutter
Picture Research Harriet Mills
Creative Technical Support Sonia Charbonnier
Production Controller James Carey
Art Director Peter Luff
Publisher Stephanie Jackson

Project Editor Louise Frances
Designer Ruth Hope
Illustrator André Metzger

First American Edition, 2008
This edition published 2010

Published in the United States by
DK Publishing
375 Hudson Street
New York, New York 10014

10 11 12 13 10 9 8 7 6 5 4 3 2 1
RD160—September 2010

Published in Great Britain by Dorling Kindersley Limited.

A catalog record for this book is available from the
Library of Congress.
ISBN 978-0-7566-5990-5

DK books are available at special discounts when purchased in bulk
for sales promotions, premiums, fund-raising, or educational use. For
details, contact: DK Publishing Special Markets, 375 Hudson Street,
New York, New York 10014 or SpecialSales@dk.com.

Color reproduction by MDP, Bath, UK
Printed and bound in Singapore by Tien Wah Press

Discover more at **www.dk.com**

This book is dedicated to my grandma, Teal Friedman, who has
always been unequivocally supportive of me, and my choices, and
who gets more gorgeous and sexy every year. Happy 90th birthday!

Author Acknowledgments

A special thank you to Dorling Kindersley Publishing, especially
Stephanie Jackson, Nichole Morford, and Louise Frances, as well
as to my phenomenal agent, Binky Urban, for embracing the vision
of this book and for your willingness to take real sex to real women!
I feel so lucky to be working with all of you. Thank you also to
Empower Public Relations for working so tirelessly and creatively
on my behalf as well as my managers at Roar, Greg Suess and Erik
Stone. And to Bridget Sharkey, I am so grateful to you for helping
me put my thoughts into words every day. This book wouldn't have
been possible without you. Thank you for understanding me so well
and for always taking my voice to the next level.

Thank you to all the women in my life for your support and for
reminding me not to take myself, or life, too seriously. To my Mom,
Linda Berman, thank you for teaching me from so early on about
being open and real. I may complain sometimes, but I love and
appreciate the honesty with which you live your life and strive to do
the same. And to my dad, Irwin Berman, thank you teaching me
that if you do what you love, then the rest will follow and for living
your life by that example.

To my amazing Sam, thank you for all you do for our family and
for me. Without your insights, support, and love this book and so
many other things wouldn't be possible. And to our three magical
boys, Ethan, Sammy, and Jackson, you always remind me of what's
important. I love you oodles and oodles of noodles.

DK Acknowledgments

Adam Brackenbury and John Goldsmid for retouching work.
Ally Williams for fabulous on-set attention to make-up and hair, and
Eleanor Hicks for assisting with prop styling. Marie Lorimer for
indexing, and Astella Saw for proofreading. Kesta Desmond, John
Windell, Jo Godfrey Wood, and Anne Johnson for their invaluable help
with editorial. Myla, for supplying "Forget Me Knot" shown on pp. 187
and 189 (Inquiries: www.myla.com and 212.327.2676).

Picture Credits

The publisher would like to thank the following for their kind
permission to reproduce their photographs:
(Key: a-above; b-below/bottom; c-centre; l-left; r-right; t-top)
25 PunchStock: Image Source (tl). 33 Science Photo Library: Helen
Mcardle. 37 PunchStock: PhotoAlto Agency. 41 PunchStock: Digital
Vision/ Helen McArdle. 43 PunchStock: Digital Vision/Adam Gault.
44 SuperStock: age fotostock. 49 Getty Images: Stone/Ebby May.
53 PunchStock: Cultura/ Philip Lee Harvey. 67 Getty Images: Stone/
Loungepark. 68 PunchStock: Image Source. 79 Getty Images: The
Image Bank/Michael Poehlman. 93 PunchStock: Blend Images/JGI.
126 Photolibrary: Photographer's Choice/ Simon Stanmore. 192
PunchStock: UpperCut Images/Hill Creek Pictures. 197 Alamy
Images: Tony Rusecki. 199 Getty Images: Photographer's Choice/Piotr
Powietrzynski. 202 Getty Images: altrendo images. 205 Getty Images:
Stone+/Javier Pierini. 221 PunchStock: Digital Vision. 225
PunchStock: Stockbyte. 230 Photolibrary: OJO Images/Paul Bradbury.

All other images © Dorling Kindersley
For further information see: www.dkimages.com